The Essential Guide to Problem Substance Use During Pregnancy

A resource book for professionals

The Essential Guide to Problem Substance Use During Pregnancy
A resource book for professionals

Published by
DrugScope
Prince Consort House (Suite 204)
109–111 Farringdon Road
London EC1R 3BW
E-mail: info@drugscope.org.uk
Website: www.drugscope.org.uk

First published by NHS Lothian 2003: 'Substance misuse in pregnancy: a resource pack for professionals in Lothian'.

Published by DrugScope 2005: 'Substance misuse in pregnancy: a resource book for professionals'.

This updated edition DrugScope 2011

Written by Anne Whittaker
Nurse Facilitator (Drugs/Alcohol/BBV),
Primary Care Facilitator Team, NHS Lothian.

DrugScope is the national membership organisation for the drug sector and a leading drug information and policy charity. **DrugScope** has over 600 members working in the drug sector and related fields and the organisation draws on the expertise of its members to develop policy and lobby government.

ISBN: 978 1 904319 53 5

Design: Helen Joubert Design

Printed in England by CPI Antony Rowe, Chippenham, Wiltshire

Contents

The appendices of this book are also available as downloadable leaflets. To access the documents please visit www.drugscope.org.uk/pregnancyguide. Please note that while printing and photocopying the appendices is permitted, they remain copyrighted to DrugScope ©2011.

Acknowledgements

Many professionals contributed to, supported and offered constructive comments on the original edition of this resource book, and on this latest edition. They include midwives, obstetricians, neonatal nurses, neonatologists, health visitors, paediatricians, general practitioners, pharmacists, drug specialists, alcohol specialists, blood borne virus specialists, public health staff, dental hospital staff, social work and voluntary sector staff.

Anne would specifically like to thank the following people for their input: Pauline Connelly and all the Link Midwives and Link Health Visitors for Substance Misuse, Karla Napier and all the Infant Feeding Advisors, Dr Rhona Hughes, Dr Sarah Cooper, Dr Paula Midgley, Anne Neilson, Jane Henry, Breda Wilson, Dr Jacqueline Mok, Dr Helen Hammond, Dr Aysel Crocket, Jenny Carson, Sherry Wright, Elaine Rankine, Dr Gordon Scott, Dr Andrew Bathgate, Dr Kate Templeton, Dr Muriel Simmonte, Dr Ewen Stewart, Dr David Ewart, Euan MacLeay, Dr Catriona Morton, Dr Fiona Watson, Dr Judith Craven, Debbie Eccles, Jim Shanley, Dr Alison McCallum, Jim Sherval, Michelle McCoy, Graham MacKenzie, Dr Jonathan Chick, Eleanor McWhirter, Chris Cunningham, Michele Kirkpatrick, Joyce Leggate, Faye Macrory and Dr Mary Hepburn.

Finally, a special thanks to all the service users (mothers and fathers) who contributed to the development of the service user information leaflets.

Introduction

Welcome to *The Essential Guide to Problem Substance Use During Pregnancy*, a resource book for professionals.

Many different professionals and agencies are now involved in the care of women who use drugs and/or alcohol during the course of their reproductive life. All professionals have an equally important role to play in ensuring a high standard of care is delivered. *The Essential Guide to Problem Substance Use During Pregnancy* aims to establish a 'framework for care' so that all women who use substances can be offered appropriate support before, during and after the birth of their child.

The framework for care consists of a philosophy of approach and good practice guidance, underpinned by evidence-based information and advice. The framework for care outlined in the book, provides a basis from which the best possible outcomes can be achieved for mother, baby and family.

A broad view of drug use is taken that includes alcohol and nicotine. This is because the risks of these drugs in pregnancy are well established and they are often used in combination with illicit, prescribed or 'over the counter' drugs. Having said this, the book refers mainly to the care of women who have significant problems related to drug and alcohol use. This is because social and lifestyle factors often complicate the delivery of care to these women. Their care often provides the biggest challenge for professionals and much co-ordination and understanding between services is needed.

Terminology

The terminology used in this resource book has been carefully chosen so as to avoid language that implies value judgements or has negative connotations. For instance, the terms *drug and alcohol dependence*, *drug and alcohol related problems*, *drug use*, *problem drinking* or *problem substance use* are used in preference to terms such as *addiction*, *drug addict*, *alcoholic*, *drug habit*, *drug misuse* and *drug abuse*. The use of currently preferred terminology is especially important when working with substance-using parents who often feel stigmatised and are sensitive to negative professional judgements.

Definitions

Problem drug use

The Advisory Council on the Misuse of Drugs (ACMD 2003) defines 'problem drug use' in *Hidden Harm* as any drug use which has serious negative consequences of a physical, psychological, social and interpersonal, financial or legal nature for users and those around them. They state that such drug use is normally heavy, with features of dependence, and typically involves the use of one or more of the following drugs: opiates (e.g. heroin and methadone); benzodiazepines (e.g. diazepam); and stimulants (e.g. crack cocaine and amphetamines).

Problem alcohol use

Three types of problem drinking have been defined (SIGN 2003): 'hazardous drinking', 'harmful drinking' and 'alcohol dependence'.

Hazardous drinking refers to the regular consumption of:
- over 40 g of pure ethanol (5 units or more) per day for *men, or* more than the recommended weekly limit (i.e. >21 units for men).
- over 24 g of pure ethanol (3 units or more) per day for *women*[1], or more than the recommended weekly limit (i.e. >14 units for women).

Hazardous drinking also includes **'binge drinking'** which is defined as excessive consumption of alcohol on any one occasion involving 8 units or more for men, and 6 units or more for women[1], even though they may not exceed weekly limits.

Harmful drinking is defined in the International Classification of Diseases (ICD-10 criteria, WHO 1992) as a pattern of drinking that causes damage to physical or mental health. The diagnosis requires that actual damage should have been caused to the physical or mental health of the user. Harmful drinking also includes drinking at levels that may be causing substantial harm to others (HM Government 2007).

---

1 Pertains to women who are not pregnant, breastfeeding or trying to conceive.

Drug and alcohol dependence

'Drug/alcohol dependence' is classed as a syndrome and defined in the International Classification of Diseases (ICD-10 criteria, WHO 1992) as 'a cluster of behavioural, cognitive and physiological phenomena that develop after repeated substance use', and typically includes:

- a strong desire to take the substance
- a higher priority given to substance use than to other activities and obligations
- difficulties controlling its use
- persisting in its use despite harmful consequences
- increased tolerance to the substance
- a physical withdrawal state.

Normally, a diagnosis of drug/alcohol dependence is made when three or more of the above criteria have been experienced or exhibited in the previous year. Distinctions are sometimes made between 'psychological' and 'physical' dependence in order to call attention to different characteristics of the syndrome (Department of Health 2007a). Relapse (or reinstatement of problem drinking or drug-taking after a period of abstinence) is a common feature.

Sources of literature and evidence

The information and guidance in this book are based on current best practice and available evidence. Sources include: governmental policy documents, contemporary social theory and health care practice, good practice guidance, clinical guidelines, expert opinion and recent publications from experienced practitioners in the field as well as a journal and publications search.

The book is not fully referenced but those references that are cited are recommended for further reading. Other helpful sources of information, addresses and websites are included. A glossary provides definitions of terms.

The book is not designed to be read cover to cover, but it is worth taking a little time to familiarise yourself with the layout and content so that you can access information easily when you need to. It is worthwhile reading the 'key points' and 'philosophy of approach' before other sections.

Key points

Most pregnant women with problem substance use will have a normal pregnancy, labour, delivery and a full-term normal birth-weight baby. Most will embrace motherhood and family life and will want to do the best for their children.

Many conditions carry with them an element of risk or uncertainty during pregnancy and require greater care. Increased risks are associated with tobacco, alcohol and drug use during pregnancy. Professionals and agencies should work together to offer information, advice, treatment and care that will help reduce these risks.

Maternal and neonatal outcomes are poorer for women from disadvantaged, vulnerable and marginalised groups. Severe drug and alcohol problems are closely associated with poverty, social deprivation, violence, criminal behaviour, poor health and social exclusion. Families affected by problem substance use often have complex health and social problems and additional needs that require an enhanced response from health and social services.

Philosophy of approach

- Many factors affect pregnancy outcome and the health and development of infants and children. Problem substance use is just one factor. A *holistic* assessment and package of care needs to be offered. The woman's lifestyle and social circumstances, her physical and psychological needs, her parenting support needs, as well as the needs of her unborn child should be taken into account.

- Engaging with *fathers* and involving them in all aspects of the care process is vital. Research shows that fathers can play an important role (both positive and negative) in the health and wellbeing of the mother during pregnancy, the care of the newborn infant, and the life-long wellbeing and development of the child, regardless of whether the father is resident or not.

- The approach taken by professionals is a crucial factor in the delivery and outcome of care. Pregnant women with problem substance use are subject to social disapproval and judgemental attitudes. Discriminatory professional practice deters women from seeking help. Professionals need to encourage women to engage with helping agencies and ensure that their approach to care is based on good evidence and best practice.

- The guiding principle of management should be a *pragmatic* approach that emphasises *harm reduction, recovery* and *social integration* and aims to achieve the best possible outcome for mother, baby and family. This means taking account of the parent's wishes, recognising their strengths and resources, as well as their vulnerabilities and needs, and focusing on what *could* be done rather than what *should* be done.

- A well co-ordinated *multi-disciplinary* and *inter-agency* approach will ensure that a comprehensive package of care can be offered. All professionals involved in the woman and infant's care, need to communicate with one another to ensure that they share a common approach, offer consistent advice and are working towards the same goals. Equally, professionals working with fathers/partners, carers (e.g. kinship carers), and other children living in the household, need to ensure that they are actively involved in the care planning process so that a 'whole family' approach is achieved.

Pre-conception care

- Agencies in contact with women and men who use substances should routinely enquire if they plan to have children. All agencies have a part to play in offering pre-conception advice and care.
- Discuss family planning, safer sex, the use of condoms, contraception methods, and fertility issues with both men and women substance users.
- Specialist pre-conception advice and support regarding substance use might include: blood borne virus testing, smoking cessation advice and support, brief interventions to reduce alcohol consumption, illicit (street) drug use and injecting, reviewing drug/alcohol treatment plans and medications.

Antenatal care

- Late presentation and poor attendance for antenatal care is associated with poor pregnancy and infant outcomes, irrespective of continued substance use. All pregnant women with problem substance use and their partners should be told about the benefits of antenatal care and encouraged to attend early in pregnancy.
- Specific information about the effects of drugs (including tobacco and alcohol) during pregnancy should be routinely given to all women identified as having

problem substance use. Likewise, the risks associated with paternal substance use should be discussed.

- Drug dependent women and their partners should be given information and advice about Neonatal Abstinence Syndrome (NAS) and the special care that their infant might need. All carers of babies with NAS should be trained in the use of supportive comfort measures. Likewise, alcohol dependent women and their partners should be given information and advice about Fetal Alcohol Syndrome (FAS) and the special care that their infant might need.
- Breastfeeding should be promoted (unless the woman is HIV positive), and the benefits of breastfeeding should be discussed early in pregnancy.
- Postnatal contraception should be discussed and agreed *before* delivery.

Assessing needs and risks during pregnancy
- Professionals should undertake a continuous risk assessment throughout pregnancy to identify any problems that could affect the mother, her pregnancy and the wellbeing of the baby.
- Emphasis should be placed on ensuring an assessment of the family's needs is undertaken during pregnancy and a *family support plan* is in place well before the baby is born.
- Assessing and improving the family's home and social circumstances during the antenatal period will help to promote the health and wellbeing of mother, baby and family.
- Problem substance use is not sufficient reason *in itself*, to assume that parenting or child care will be inadequate. However, parental problem substance use is associated with an increased risk of poor parenting capacity, poor child development and increased rates of child maltreatment. Infants affected by Neonatal Abstinence Syndrome and Fetal Alcohol Syndrome have special care needs. Young infants in particular are extremely vulnerable to the negative effects of abuse and neglect. The safety and welfare of the newborn baby is paramount and professionals should follow child protection procedures if 'significant harm' is likely.

Management of substance use during pregnancy
- Pregnant women and prospective fathers with problem substance use should be given priority access to drug and alcohol treatment services. Treatment goals should be realistic and achievable and tailored to their individual needs.

- Pregnancy and the early postnatal period is a time when mothers and fathers are often willing to discuss their aspirations and lifestyle and may be more receptive to harm reduction and health improvement interventions, especially where there is a proven benefit to the baby.
- Professionals should discuss a range of treatment options with mothers and fathers, including: smoking cessation interventions, alcohol brief interventions, safer injecting techniques, reducing illicit drug use, stabilising dependent drug use, drug dose reduction, detoxification, relapse prevention, abstinence, psychological therapies and social support programmes.
- Pregnant drug users and their partners should not be pressurised into coming off drugs. This can lead to more harm than good, especially if the parents disengage from services.

Intrapartum care
- Although most women with problem substance use will have a normal labour and delivery, they often do need help to prepare for hospital admission. Opiate dependent women should be reassured that they will be given adequate pain relief during childbirth.
- Fathers should be encouraged to take an active role in the care and support of the mother during labour and delivery.
- Following delivery, parents should care for their baby in the postnatal ward. Separating mother and baby should be avoided wherever possible. As with all women, they should be encouraged to breastfeed, bond and care for their baby.

Postnatal care
- Parents with problem substance use may need considerable help and support with parenthood and child care. Parents with other children to look after may need more support not less. Planned support that continues well into the postnatal period is crucial.
- A strengths-based approach which aims to enhance parenting capacity, and interventions which target couples and families rather than parents as individuals, are most effective.
- Multi-disciplinary discharge planning should aim to ensure that the infant is cared for in a safe and nurturing environment. Infants with NAS may have delayed growth and development for several months. Children with FAS may have life long developmental needs. Parents often need additional support to

foster secure attachments, to improve parent-infant interactions, and to ensure developmental issues are addressed.

- The postnatal period can be a very stressful time for parents. For mothers and fathers who have managed to reduce their substance use during the antenatal period, the risk of relapse to former levels and patterns of substance use is high. Relapse prevention work, careful substance use management, psychosocial interventions and intensive structured family support may be required for some time.

Setting the scene

The extent of the problem

The true extent of drug taking in women is largely unknown as reliable figures are hard to obtain (NTA 2010). It is clear, however, that smoking, alcohol use and illicit drug use in women of reproductive age is widespread and the continued use of drugs during pregnancy is common. Approximately 33% of women smoke during pregnancy (NHS Information Centre 2007) and 54% consume alcohol during pregnancy, albeit at low levels predominantly (NHS Information Centre 2010). The use of illicit drugs during pregnancy such as cannabis, amphetamines, heroin and cocaine is thought to be moderately prevalent, especially in large urban areas. For many women, substance use is a fundamental part of their lives.

Although nicotine and alcohol are legally available it is important not to confuse legality with safety. Maternal use of tobacco is well researched and known to have significant harmful effects on pregnancy (NICE 2008a). Although approximately 48% of women who smoke manage to give up at some stage during pregnancy, nicotine remains the most problematic drug of use at a population level (Johnstone 1998), with 27% of pregnant women in the UK reporting that they are current smokers at the time of the birth of the baby (NICE 2008a). Alcohol has the clearest association with teratogenesis (congenital birth defects), with well-documented adverse effects associated with high maternal intake (RCOG 2006, BMA 2007a). Approximately 30% of women of reproductive age exceed the recommended weekly limit of alcohol consumption (RCM 2010, Scottish Government 2009a). Nicotine and alcohol are often used in combination with other drugs and most women who present to drug and alcohol treatment services report 'polydrug use'.

The nature of the problem

Many factors affect the outcome of pregnancy and the health and wellbeing of mother and baby. Many conditions carry with them an element of risk or uncertainty and require greater care during pregnancy. Substance use is just one factor. Other factors include lifestyle and social circumstances, physical and psychological health, nutrition, breastfeeding, sexually transmitted and communicable diseases, antenatal and postnatal care. The involvement and support of the father/woman's partner and the wider family and community is also a key issue.

Women who seek help for alcohol and drug related problems are more likely to be unemployed and living in areas of social deprivation. Many report a history of childhood abuse and/or neglect, and are from excluded, vulnerable or marginalised groups (Best & Abdulrahim 2005). Pregnant women with problem substance use and their partners often present with multiple and complex needs that require the involvement of many different professionals and agencies. The organisation and delivery of care therefore, is an important factor in outcome (Johnstone 1998, Moran *et al* 2009).

Organisational difficulties

Professionals who are experienced in working with this client group often report a number of problems. These include:

- No common or 'shared' approach to care
- Lack of understanding of professional roles and responsibilities
- Little consultation or 'joined-up' assessment process
- Limited 'partnership' of care with the woman
- Little engagement or involvement of the father/partner
- Unrealistic expectations and treatment goals
- Inconsistent and contradictory advice
- Difficulty organising inter-agency care plan meetings or reviews
- Poor liaison and communication between professionals
- No one professional taking responsibility for co-ordinating care.

For midwives, delivering care to this client group can be very time consuming. Committed midwives can often spend considerable time co-ordinating care, liaising with other professionals, organising antenatal and postnatal care planning meetings, organising the additional antenatal care requirements that these women often need, and visiting in excess of 10 days postpartum.

In addition to organisational and service delivery difficulties there are a number of other reasons why the care of pregnant women with drug and/or alcohol related problems has been difficult for health and social care providers.

Ideology

The prevailing societal view of women with problem substance use is a negative one. Alcohol and drug dependent women have been characterised as irresponsible, inadequate, deviant, immoral and unfit for motherhood. Research shows that women who are alcohol or drug dependent get significantly more social disapproval than men (Klee *et al* 2002, Ehrmin 2001). In pregnancy, this view is heightened as the welfare of the unborn child is emphasised and assumptions are made about the harmful consequences of the mother's drug/alcohol use and her ability to be a 'good mother' and care adequately for her child (Macrory & Crosby 1995, Lester *et al* 2004). This gender bias has led to punitive responses, unacceptable levels of scrutiny and surveillance and restricted options for treatment and care (Lester *et al* 2004, ACOG 2008). Negative societal views and professional attitudes coupled with discriminatory practice have deterred women from seeking help (Klee *et al* 2002, ACOG 2008). Some pregnant women may appear to neglect their condition and that of their babies but in reality it may be the service's negative attitudes and hostile approach that have excluded them from care (Lester *et al* 2004).

Fathers with drug and alcohol problems are also viewed negatively (Klee 1998, McMahon & Giannini 2003). Often they are characterised as absent or uninvolved fathers, who are unconcerned about the welfare of the mother, and pose a threat to the safety and wellbeing of the infant. Research shows that disadvantaged, marginalised and young fathers, tend to be unsupported and ignored by professionals, despite the men being a potential asset and/or a potential risk to the family (Lewis & Lamb 2007, Daniel & Taylor 2001). A focus on fathers and fatherhood in recent years, along with the 'Think Family' approach to parenting interventions, and legislation on equality and diversity, has drawn attention to these important issues around the time of childbirth (Fatherhood Institute 2010).

Lack of good quality research evidence

Lack of good quality research on the effects of alcohol and drug use on the fetus and baby has led to some confusion and exaggeration of risk (Lester *et al* 2004). Few studies take into account multiple confounding factors that are known to influence pregnancy and infant outcomes (Kaltenbach 1994, Schempf 2007). Good quality studies on the medical management of pregnant women and infants affected by substance use are also lacking (Lester *et al* 2004, Winklbaur *et al* 2008, NICE 2010a). Research reviews tend to only deal with one aspect of the overall presenting problem, making evidence-based management particularly challenging (Winklbaur *et al* 2008). Providing balanced and factual information to women so that they can make informed choices during pregnancy has proved difficult, and women continue to receive inconsistent and contradictory advice.

Equally, the impact of *paternal* substance use on pregnancy and infant outcomes is often overlooked and is under-researched (Frank *et al* 2002, McMahon & Rounsaville 2002, McMahon *et al* 2008). What is clear is that outcomes for mothers, babies and families affected by problem substance use are multi-factorial, influenced by a dynamic interplay of individual, social, psychosocial, behavioural, biological, legal, economic and organisational factors. An 'ecological approach' (Department of Health 2000) to understanding and responding to pregnant women and families affected by problem substance use should therefore be adopted.

Women's fears

Not surprisingly, pregnant women substance users frequently report a number of concerns including:
- Fear of being automatically referred to social services
- Fear that her baby will be taken into care
- Fear and confusion over whether her substance use will cause fetal damage
- Fear that she will be blamed if anything goes wrong with her pregnancy
- Fear of being thought of as an uncaring or 'unfit' mother if she doesn't manage to come off or reduce her drug use
- Feeling guilty and 'to blame' for her baby experiencing withdrawal symptoms.

Poor social circumstances

Drug and alcohol related problems are commonly associated with poverty, deprivation and poor social circumstances (Shaw *et al* 2007). These include:
- Lack of support from family and friends
- Poor support from a substance-using partner
- Substance related criminal activity and legal problems (e.g. outstanding charges, impending court cases, community service order, probation, prison history, drug treatment and testing orders)
- Current or past history of sexual abuse/exploitation
- Violence and intimidation (e.g. substance-related or domestic abuse)

- Financial problems (including debts, fines and problems with welfare benefits)
- Housing problems (including homelessness, insecure or unsuitable housing)
- Lack of education and training and employability problems (such as no qualifications or skills, poor work performance, poor sick leave record, long term unemployment).

Maternal health problems

Injecting drug use, unstable drug use and harmful levels of drinking are associated with poor maternal health. This may include:

- Poor diet (including malnutrition and anaemia)
- Respiratory problems
- Poor dental hygiene
- Blood borne virus infections (HIV, hepatitis B, hepatitis C)
- Complications from injecting (such as abscesses, endocarditis, septicaemia etc)
- Liver disease
- Accidental injury
- Overdose and maternal death
- Mental health problems (such as anxiety, depression, self harm, psychosis)
- Poor sexual health.

Lifestyle issues

Drug and alcohol related problems are commonly associated with a disorganised or unconventional lifestyle which lacks normal daily routines and adherence to everyday activities and obligations. This may result in the woman not attending appointments and the woman receiving poor maternity care. For example:

- Late pregnancy booking
- Poor attendance for antenatal care
- Not registering with a general practitioner
- Poor attendance for parenthood education
- Late presentation during labour
- Early discharge home after delivery
- Failure to attend child health appointments.

Obstetric and paediatric problems

Drug use (including tobacco and alcohol) impacts on obstetric and paediatric morbidity and mortality. Increased rates of low birth weight, preterm delivery, Sudden Infant Death Syndrome (SIDS or 'cot death'), Neonatal Abstinence Syndrome (NAS) and Fetal Alcohol Syndrome (FAS) are the most commonly reported problems (Johnstone 1998, Hepburn 2004a, BMA 2007a, Moran *et al* 2009). Information on the effects of specific substances on the developing fetus and baby are outlined later in this book.

It is well established that many obstetric problems associated with problem drug and alcohol use are also associated with poverty, social deprivation, social exclusion, poor maternal health and nutrition, maternal and paternal smoking, and poor antenatal care (Department of Health 2007a, NICE 2010a). A number of case controlled studies have found comparable pregnancy outcomes in women (who are matched by age, parity, social deprivation category etc) who do not have substance use problems (Kaltenbach 1994, Siney 1999).

Some obstetric outcomes (e.g. low birth weight and preterm delivery) are now considered indicators for tackling health and social inequalities. Birth weight of less than 2.5 kg is associated with poor child health and delayed physical and intellectual development (Department of Health 2004a). Risk of infant death is almost 2.5 times greater, and risk of maternal death in the year following birth is almost 5 times more likely, if living in an area of deprivation (CEMACH 2007). Women with complex social factors tend to book later than other women, and late booking is associated with poor obstetric and neonatal outcomes (NICE 2010a). Social and contextual factors, including the quality of health and social care provision, significantly influence the health and wellbeing of both mother and baby (CEMACH 2007, NICE 2010a).

Because of such complications, problem substance use during pregnancy has become one of the leading conditions requiring specific guidelines and strategies.

The next section outlines guiding principles that form a 'framework for care'.

Framework for care

There are several publications which provide a broad set of principles, and guidance on good practice, for working with pregnant women and families affected by alcohol and drug problems. In the UK, devolved responsibility for health and social care means that these publications are not necessarily applicable across the whole of England, Wales, Scotland and Northern Ireland. Nevertheless, these documents are largely consistent and/or complementary and do offer valuable key messages for practice. A selection is included below:

Maternity and Early Years guidance includes:
- *Maternity and Early Years – making a good start to family life* (HM Government 2010)
- *Maternity Services: National Service Framework for children, young people and maternity services* (DfES and Department of Health 2004)
- *Maternity Matters: choice, access and continuity of care in a safe service* (Department of Health 2007)
- *Getting maternity services right for pregnant teenagers and young fathers* (DCSF & Department of Health 2009)
- *The Child Health Promotion Programme: Pregnancy and first five years of life* (DCSF and Department of Health 2008)
- *Every Child Matters: change for children* (HM Government 2004)
- *Every Parent Matters* (DfES 2007)
- *Think Family: improving the life chances of families at risk* (Cabinet Office 2008)
- *A Framework for Maternity Services in Scotland* (Scottish Executive 2001)
- *Clinical Standards: Maternity Services* (NHSQIS 2005)
- *Enhanced maternity services for women within NHS Scotland* (Scottish Government 2009)
- *Getting it right for every child – GIRFEC* (Scottish Executive 2005)
- *The Early Years Framework* (Scottish Government 2008)
- *Royal College of Midwives* (RCM) and *Royal College of Obstetricians and Gynaecologists* (RCOG) clinical guidelines and position statements.

Drug and alcohol specific guidance includes:

- *Drug misuse and dependence: UK guidelines on clinical management* (Department of Health 2007)
- *Drugs: protecting families and communities* (HM Government 2008)
- *Drug strategy 2010 – reducing demand, restricting supply, building recovery* (HM Government 2010)
- *Safe, Sensible, Social: the next steps in the National Alcohol Strategy* (HM Government 2007)
- *The road to recovery: a new approach to tackling Scotland's drug problem* (Scottish Government 2008)
- *Changing Scotland's relationship with alcohol: a framework for action* (Scottish Government 2009)
- *Working together to reduce harm: the substance misuse strategy for Wales 2008–2018* (Welsh Assembly Government 2008)
- *New strategic direction for alcohol and drugs 2006–2011* (DHSSPS Northern Ireland 2006)
- *Hidden Harm: responding to the needs of children of problem drug users* (ACMD 2003)
- *Getting our priorities right: good practice guidance for working with children and families affected by substance misuse* (Scottish Executive 2003)

Philosophy of approach

The philosophy of approach outlined here reflects the central themes from these policy documents and clinical guidelines as well as recommendations from leading experts in the field.

Overall, the approach to care needs to be:
- women-centred and family-orientated
- non-judgemental and non-discriminatory
- pragmatic, with an emphasis on harm reduction and social integration
- holistic, based on an ecological model of family functioning and human development
- focussed on ensuring the safety and wellbeing of the infant
- provided by a multi-disciplinary team, involving inter-agency working.

Women-centred and family-orientated approach

Pregnancy and the transition into parenthood is a significant life event. For women who have problems related to alcohol or drug use it offers opportunities as well as risks. These women have the same hopes and aspirations for family life and the same anxieties about pregnancy, childbirth and motherhood as other women (Hepburn 2004). For service providers, the challenge is to offer the right kind of support at the right time to allow them to minimise the risks as much as possible and to make the most of available opportunities. This means that treatment and care needs to be women-centred and family-orientated (RCM 2008a, HM Government 2010a).

The important role of partners needs to be recognised, and professionals need to ensure that, where appropriate, they are encouraged and supported to take a full and active role in pregnancy, the birth and postnatal child care (DfES 2007, HM Government 2010a). Women and their partners need to be able to make fully informed choices about their care. They need timely, relevant and easily accessible information to help them make the choices they face. They also need prompt access to any treatment and care that they might need.

Maternity care should be tailored to the needs of the individual woman and her family, focusing on the safety of mother and baby. It should take into account:

- the needs and wishes of the woman and her family
- her right to privacy and dignity throughout her pregnancy
- her cultural values, beliefs, attitudes, and chosen lifestyle.

A family-orientated approach will create an atmosphere of normalisation and partnership that will engage the woman and her partner and foster the best possible outcome for mother, baby and family.

Non-judgemental and non-discriminatory approach

Service providers need to adopt a truly professional approach that is not led by views which are distorted by prejudice or limited by conventional stereotypes (Klee et al 2002). Professionals need to continually examine their approach to care so that they can account for their practice in terms of what is in the best interests of the woman and her baby and what is in accordance with the best available evidence and best practice.

Establishing early contact with pregnant women who have substance use problems, retaining them in treatment and care, and providing them with the right kind of care is vital (Department of Health 2007a, NICE 2010a). This can best be achieved by creating a supportive, culturally sensitive and non-discriminatory environment. Providing care with compassion, empathy and encouragement will facilitate good contact. A non-judgemental approach is also a pre-requisite for obtaining the necessary details of the woman's substance use, the partner's substance use and their social circumstances. The woman and her partner need to feel supported throughout the pregnancy and beyond. This means that professionals need to create a positive pregnancy experience for the prospective parents, irrespective of risk and despite any difficulties that they may face.

Pragmatic approach

Substance use during pregnancy is associated with increased risks. Pregnancy therefore provides an excellent opportunity for professionals to provide education and care within a harm reduction framework (Johnstone 1998, Department of Health 2007a, Moran *et al* 2009). Harm reduction is a pragmatic approach to care which aims to reduce the harm to individuals and society whether or not it is possible to reduce the substance use *per se* (O'Hare *et al* 1992). It is essentially a public health policy designed to minimise risk. It is a reality-based approach that focuses on what *could* be done rather than what *should* be done. A harm reduction approach includes providing the means, information and education to enable people to make informed choices about their lifestyle.

Treatment and care goals must be realistic and achievable and tailored to the needs of the individual woman (Hepburn 2004b). Pressurising pregnant women into reducing or coming off drugs may result in more harm than good (Winklbaur *et al* 2008). A flexible service that is able to take account of the wishes of the woman and support her to make her own decisions and be guided by what she feels she can achieve, will be most successful (Johnstone 1998, Moran *et al* 2009).

It is important to remember that a harm reduction approach incorporates efforts to promote social integration and recovery and includes abstinence. Abstinence can be helpfully thought of as the 'final goal' of harm reduction and one which many people with substance use problems may wish to achieve in the short term, or in the longer term. However, drug and alcohol dependence is considered a chronic relapsing condition (WHO 1992). People may use alcohol and drugs in potentially harmful ways for many years before achieving abstinence. Long-term support to help people minimise the harm associated with substance use is normally required and may include: substitute prescribing; needle exchange; psychosocial interventions, and safer drug use/sensible drinking advice and support (Robertson 1998). All these interventions can be seen as part of a person's recovery in, and from, problem substance use.

Holistic approach

Pregnant women with substance use problems often present with multiple and complex needs (NICE 2010a). Their substance use is just one aspect of their lives. A holistic approach to care, from preconception to parenthood, needs to be offered (Hepburn 2004a).

An ecological assessment should aim to identify the woman's physical, psychological and social needs, and should aim to understand her current circumstances within a relational and social/environmental context – for example, by taking into account her social support networks and socio-economic circumstances. An ecological assessment encompasses historical factors, the context and causes of any presenting problems, and considers the circumstances and needs of the whole family (Department of Health 2000, DfES 2006). It also involves identifying protective factors, resilience and the strengths, resources, knowledge and skills of the woman and her family (RCM 2008a, Scottish Executive 2005).

A holistic package of care recognises that a woman's needs are inter-related and context-dependent, and aims to provide a service that can address not just one aspect of her care, but the needs of the whole family. Strengths-based models of intervention are known to be effective (Moran *et al* 2004, Cabinet Office 2008). This involves identifying strengths and stressors in the individual, the family and the environment, and then assisting to promote the strengths and decrease the stressors.

Safeguarding the infant

Protecting a newborn infant from harm should be the paramount concern of all professionals and agencies involved in the family's care. Parental problem substance use is associated with an increased risk of poor parenting capacity, poor child development, and increased rates of child maltreatment (Cleaver *et al* 2010, ACMD 2003, Scottish Executive 2003a, WHO 2006). Parental substance use is a key contributing factor in the lives of children involved in child protection services and serious case reviews (Forrester & Harwin 2006, Forrester 2007, Brandon *et al* 2008, 2009). It should be remembered that drug and alcohol related problems are far more prevalent in men than women, and *paternal* substance use is also clearly associated with poor outcomes for children (Ornoy *et al* 1996, Frank *et al* 2002, McMahon *et al* 2002, 2008, WHO 2006). Professionals and agencies should work together to ensure that the parenting capacity of *both* parents is optimised so that they are able to provide a safe and nurturing environment for their infant.

Young infants in particular, are very vulnerable to the negative effects of abuse and/or neglect. Often babies born to mothers who are dependent on alcohol and/or drugs have special care needs in the first few days, weeks and months. This might be because the infant is born preterm, very low birth weight, or develops Neonatal Abstinence Syndrome (NAS). Babies affected by maternal alcohol use may have long term developmental and education needs on account of intellectual and neurological impairments (RCOG 2006, BMA 2007, RCM 2010).

The anticipated needs of the newborn infant should be an integral part of the assessment and care process. During the antenatal period, parenting education should focus on the mother and father's ability to prepare for parenthood and to meet the developmental needs of the child.

Multi-disciplinary and inter-agency working

Pregnant women whose drug or alcohol use is likely to impact on the outcome of their pregnancy will need a comprehensive service provided by a multi-disciplinary team. This service should provide consistent advice and support and continuity of care and aim to ensure safety for both mother and baby.

Many women will benefit from receiving care from a range of health and social care providers. This 'inter-agency' approach to care needs to be well co-ordinated as good communication between professionals is central to the provision of good quality care. Integrated care is where everyone involved in the provision of care has a shared philosophy of approach, knows what each other is doing and saying, and also knows what the woman herself needs and wants. Engaging with the father and involving him in all aspects of the care process is essential for promoting a good start to family life (HM Government 2010a).

A clear understanding of professional roles and responsibilities is needed to maximise the quality of care. Collaborative working should minimise the opportunities for contradictory or opinion-based advice and practice. Professionals delivering care need to have the knowledge and skills necessary for the type and level of service they provide. They should be aware of the expertise of other professionals and be prepared to draw upon that expertise where needed.

Pregnant women with substance use problems should receive the same quality of care, respect and dignity as any other pregnant woman throughout their pregnancy. The philosophy of approach outlined above and the guidelines on good practice that follow should ensure that this can be achieved.

Good practice guidance

This section of the resource book outlines good practice guidance for working with pregnant women, and their partners, who have problem substance use. It seeks to complement other existing guidance and to highlight key components of the care process.

The care process

It is important that all professionals involved with substance-using women follow a clear 'pathway of care', from pre-conception through to parenthood. A model 'care pathway' is included as a guide for practitioners (see appendix 1).

The care process involves four key stages:

1. Assessment
2. Planning
3. Service delivery
4. Review.

The main tasks in the care process are outlined below, along with a checklist of topics that are relevant to each stage of the process, many of which are covered in the course of routine health care as well as drug and alcohol treatment and social care service provision.

It is important to engage both parents in the assessment and care planning process, and to explain the care pathway and all that it entails, so that both parents understand what is involved and why, what is expected of them, and what they can expect from professionals and services. As a general rule, there should be no surprises and the woman and her partner should be treated with respect and dignity at all times.

Assessment

Assessment should be holistic and continuous throughout pregnancy (NICE 2008a). It should take into account the woman's physical and psychological health, her social circumstances, her substance use (including alcohol and tobacco), her partner's circumstances and substance use, and an assessment of need as well as an assessment of risk. In most cases, it will involve a number of different professionals contributing to the assessment process over time, including the general practitioner, midwife, obstetric and paediatric staff, the health visitor, drug and alcohol specialists, social workers and other social care/voluntary sector staff.

An assessment of **physical health needs** should include such topics as:
- Past obstetric/gynaecological history
- General health status and medical history
- Nutrition (e.g. diet, weight, anaemia)
- Dental health
- Exposure to infections (e.g. blood borne viruses, sexually transmitted infections)
- Complications from injecting (including venous access)
- Accidents or injuries
- Difficulty getting registered with GP.

An assessment of **psychological needs** should include such topics as:
- Worries or concerns about the pregnancy (e.g. fear baby will be taken into care, fear of damage to the fetus)
- Current or past anxiety related problems
- Current low mood or history of depression/self harm
- History of eating disorder (e.g. anorexia or bulimia)
- Low self esteem or self worth
- History of physical, emotional or sexual abuse
- Bereavement issues
- Woman's perception of her own circumstances, needs and coping ability.

An assessment of **social needs** should include:
- Housing situation (e.g. homelessness, insecure or unsuitable accommodation)
- Financial situation (e.g. debts, rent arrears, unpaid bills or fines)
- Legal situation (e.g. current charges, impending court cases, community service or probation orders, drug treatment and testing orders)
- Employment, training & education issues
- Relationships with partner, family, friends
- Available social support network
- Parenting capacity, including care of any existing children

- Contact with health and social care professionals or services.

An assessment of **substance use** should include the following:
- Smoking
- Alcohol use
- Illicit (street) drug use
- Injecting drug use
- Prescribed drug use
- Use of 'over the counter' medications
- Current contact with specialist drug/alcohol services
- Current treatment, care goals and progress
- Previous contact with drug/alcohol services
- Impact of substance use on mental state and behaviour/lifestyle
- Impact of drinking/drug culture environment.

Information on the effects of drugs on the developing fetus and baby, as well as the assessment and management of drug use during pregnancy is described in detail later in the book.

A **risk assessment** should include:
- Obstetric/gynaecological problems
- Past or current mental health problems
- Learning difficulties that significantly impact on parenting
- Domestic abuse/parental conflict
- Criminal justice involvement/history
- Teenage pregnancy/care leaver/asylum seeker/refugee
- Social isolation/unsupported pregnancy
- Previous history of child care concerns or current child protection involvement
- Previous baby with Neonatal Abstinence Syndrome or other serious neonatal problem e.g. congenital abnormality.

An assessment of the **partner's circumstances and substance use** should include:
- Partner's current use of tobacco, alcohol and drugs
- Partner's drug/alcohol treatment plan and progress
- Level of stability if drug dependent
- Partner's history of injecting drug use
- Blood borne virus status of partner

- Partner's past contact with health and social care agencies, including mental health services
- Partner's current employment, housing, and financial situation
- Partner's involvement with the criminal justice system
- Partner's social support network
- Partner's parenting capacity, including care of any children not currently living in household.

The assessment process should always involve a **home visit** to gauge the family's available resources/material possessions and to consider whether the home environment is suitable for a newborn baby. At the home visit, safe storage of methadone, alcohol and other drugs in the home can be discussed with the parents – see leaflet – 'Keeping children safe from alcohol and drugs in the home' (appendix 2). Often it is the health visitor who undertakes an antenatal home visit, but it can also be done by other professionals involved with the parents – for example, the midwife or social worker. Any concerns about the home environment can then be included in the care plan and steps can be taken to resolve them in advance of the birth and the baby going home.

At any time, where there is a level of concern about the welfare or safety of the (unborn) baby, a referral to social services should be made. If required, a pre-birth *child protection case conference* will be convened (normally around 28 weeks gestation), and a *child protection care plan* put in place.

In order to facilitate multi-disciplinary and multi-agency working, most areas now have **'single shared assessments'** which can be accessed by all the key professionals involved in the family's care. Shared assessments avoid duplication and facilitate information sharing and are set up as a secure electronic platform.

Care planning

Care should be planned in partnership with the parents. Care planning involves developing a 'package of care' that meets the family's needs and takes into account the views and wishes of the parents and the needs of the child. It includes what treatment and care will be provided, and by whom, as well as the desired outcomes. Care plans need to be realistic and achievable and they should include a timetable and a review date (Whittaker & McLeod 1998). A maternity care plan will be agreed after the booking appointment, and will cover the care to be provided by midwifery and obstetric services, but a further **multi-disciplinary/ inter-agency planning**

meeting should be arranged for around 24 weeks gestation. This should involve sharing relevant information about the family, making an analysis of what this means for the family, and then developing and agreeing a 'family support plan' for the end of the pregnancy, the early postnatal period and beyond.

A standard care plan or 'family support plan' might include some or all of the following:

- Antenatal care including screening tests, scans, and monitoring of fetal growth
- Smoking cessation support for mother and father
- Treatment and care of drug/alcohol problem (including realistic harm reduction goals and strategies)
- Plan to address blood borne virus prevention, testing, immunisation and treatment (if required)
- Plan to address any risks or concerns associated with parenting capacity
- Plan to attend to any psychological support needs or mental health problems
- Plan to address any social needs e.g. referral to housing and welfare benefit services, help with legal problems
- Preparation for parenthood (including parent education classes)
- Preparation for childbirth (labour and delivery)
- Preparation for Neonatal Abstinence Syndrome (if drug dependent)
- Preparation for infant feeding (support and encouragement to breastfeed)
- Plan for postnatal care (including preparations for infant and social support)
- Plan to involve the father/partner in the early postnatal care of the infant
- Plan to provide one-to-one education on child development, attachment and parent-infant interactions
- Plan to involve and support any kinship carers
- Plan to involve other professionals and referral to other agencies
- Plan for multi-disciplinary/inter-agency meeting/child protection case conference
- Arrangements to ensure a hospital discharge planning meeting is convened.

A *family support plan* should always include a **contingency plan** if circumstances change or problems arise or progress is not made within a certain time scale. This will help to reduce the need for crisis management if things don't turn out as planned.

Most areas now have standardised multi-agency care plan templates for children and families. However, a suggested format for a 'Family Support Plan' (see appendix

3) is included as a guide. Give the parents a copy of the care plan to take home so that they have the contact details of each professional/agency at hand.

Service delivery

Typically, supplementary services are required to help address the family's additional needs and to manage and overcome any difficulties. Pregnancy offers a very short time scale to arrange services and to ensure they are delivered in the right way, at the right time. It is therefore helpful if a named person or 'lead professional' is identified who can take responsibility for ensuring services are requested and delivered as detailed in the care plan.

When arranging services or making a referral to a professional or agency, it is important to include details of the estimated date of delivery of the baby, and to ensure that essential background information is included. If the need is pressing, mark the referral 'URGENT', and clearly explain why the service is required. Include contact details of key professionals involved in the family's care so that further information can be obtained easily, and the referral can be responded to quickly. Ensure the parents have given their consent to the referral being made and understand what is expected of them and how the service can help them.

Reviewing care plans

The fluctuating nature of problem drug and alcohol use means that it is important to re-assess 'need' and 'risk' at regular intervals and to review the care plan and progress of care throughout the pregnancy – for example, at antenatal appointments and drug/alcohol treatment appointments.

Women with multiple or complex health and social needs should have a care plan review every 4–6 weeks and attend a care plan review meeting if required. All parties involved in the delivery of care should be encouraged to contribute to the review by submitting a verbal or written report outlining progress.

The review process should include a discussion on the following topics:
- Implementation of the care plan and progress on each of the action points listed
- Attendance for antenatal care
- Fetal health and development
- Maternal health (including mental health)

- Current smoking/alcohol/drug use
- Attendance at specialist drug/alcohol service
- Attendance for other health care appointments (e.g. GP, health visitor or community mental health nurse)
- Attendance for social care appointments (e.g. social work, voluntary sector agencies)
- Stability of lifestyle
- Improvement in social circumstances
- Involvement and support of partner/kinship carers
- Partner's health and social circumstances, drug and alcohol use and progress with any treatment plans
- Current or potential risks
- Future needs to address
- Future goals to work towards.

Where a family support plan has been agreed and implemented successfully, the next multi-disciplinary/inter-agency meeting will be the **discharge planning meeting** held a few days after the baby is born. At this meeting a clear decision should be made as to whether or not the baby can be safely discharged home to the care of the parents. This will involve consideration of the mother and father's circumstances and progress, their demonstrated parenting skills and quality of parent-infant interactions, the condition of the baby and any special needs it might have, as well as the suitability of the home environment and level of social support.

If the infant is to be discharged home to the care of the parents, the family support plan can be revised before discharge to include any additional needs identified post birth.

Care co-ordination and care management

Many women with problem substance use and their families have multiple and complex needs and will require a 'care management' approach during pregnancy and well into the postnatal period. Pregnant women with problem substance use should have *as a minimum*: a named consultant obstetrician, midwife and health visitor, as well as a substance misuse specialist and a GP. Children and family social services, housing and welfare benefit agencies, criminal justice services, mental health services, a pharmacist, and other social care services, may also be involved in order to address the family's needs. Typically several different professionals (from adult and children's services), and more than one agency, are involved with most families. This means that a 'lead professional' should be appointed in order to take responsibility for co-ordinating all the services supporting a family, and to ensure that the care pathway is followed and the care process is fully documented, implemented and reviewed. The lead professional also ensures that the parents are well informed and take an active role in the process. This requires good liaison, communication and organisational skills to ensure a continuum of care is delivered in accordance with the agreed care plan for the family.

The role of the lead professional is often time-consuming, resource intensive and requires distinct competencies. For these reasons, most large urban areas have now developed specialist posts and multi-disciplinary teams for pregnant women with problem substance use.

Confidentiality and consent to share information

All professionals working with pregnant women who have alcohol and/or drug related problems need to work collaboratively with other professionals and agencies in order to provide good quality care. It is important to discuss 'information sharing' with the woman (and her partner) at an early stage so that informed consent can be obtained to allow joint working. Most parents are happy to agree to this once the benefits of inter-agency collaboration are explained. Information regarding the assessment, care plan and progress can then be exchanged between professionals.

Although the woman (and her partner) may consent to 'information sharing' and 'joint working' they may still need reassurance about their right to privacy and should be given information on professional 'confidentiality', the *Data Protection Act* (1998) and the *Freedom of Information Act* (2000)/ *Freedom of Information (Scotland) Act* 2002. This should include advice about circumstances whereby confidentiality may be breached and information may be shared *without* the woman or partner's consent – for example, for child protection, adult protection, mental health or legal reasons.

Guidance on confidentiality and information sharing is contained within documents such as *Inter-agency child protection procedures, Inter-agency data sharing agreements*, the *Common Assessment Framework* (CAF), *National guidance for child protection in Scotland* (Scottish Government 2010a), as well as within ethical codes of conduct published by professional bodies (e.g. Nursing and Midwifery Council) and directives issued by Chief Medical Officers. The Department for Children,

Schools and Families (DCSF 2008, now Department for Education) also published a useful guidance document for reference on-line: *Information sharing: guidance for practitioners and managers.*

Although many services now ask service users to sign 'consent forms' to allow professionals to share information about families, practitioners should be careful not to assume that service users who sign these forms agree to sharing **all** information to **all** agencies for an indefinite period of time. The principle of sharing information on a 'need to know' basis is well recognised, and it is good practice to discuss information sharing with service users **when it occurs**, and to document this clearly in the service user's notes. This will help maintain an open and honest dialogue about joint working arrangements.

Information on substance use

Ideally, all professionals who provide care to pregnant women with drug and alcohol problems should be able to:

- Provide information on the risks associated with tobacco, alcohol and drug use during pregnancy
- Assess drug and alcohol related problems during pregnancy
- Provide evidence-based advice about how to reduce harms and effectively manage problem substance use during pregnancy
- Discuss a range of options for the treatment and care of problem substance use during pregnancy.

If professionals cannot provide the above then they should ensure that they refer women to services that can.

The next section of the resource book provides information and good practice guidance on these topics.

Trends in substance use (illicit and prescribed)

This section includes basic information on commonly used drugs in the UK for professionals not familiar with illicit (non-prescribed) and prescribed drug use.

Commonly used drugs in the UK include:

- alcohol
- cannabis ('hash' and marijuana)
- benzodiazepines (e.g. diazepam, temazepam)
- opioids (e.g. heroin, methadone, dihydrocodeine, buprenorphine)
- hallucinogens (e.g. LSD or acid, 'magic mushrooms')
- stimulants (such as amphetamine, cocaine, ecstasy, mephedrone, naphyrone and other substances known as 'legal highs')
- other drugs (such as cyclizine, ketamine, gammahydroxybutrate or 'GHB', gammabutyrolactone or 'GBL', amyl nitrite or 'poppers', anabolic steroids, anti-depressants and anti-psychotics)
- volatile substances (e.g. gas, glue, and aerosols)

- over-the-counter drugs such as those containing codeine and dihydrocodeine.

Most women who use drugs do not inject them (NTA 2010). Oral 'polydrug' use is more common, although rates of injecting and oral drug use vary from one area to another and over time, and the route of administration varies depending on the type of drug used (some drugs are easier to inject than others e.g. heroin and amphetamine).

Cannabis is the most widely used illicit drug and is normally mixed with tobacco and smoked in a 'joint' or 'spliff'. Central nervous system (CNS) stimulant drugs, such as amphetamine, ecstasy, cocaine, and so-called 'legal highs' are commonly used for recreational purposes and are popular in the dance club social scene. Anti-depressants (mostly 'SSRIs') are also in widespread use. They are prescribed for the treatment of depression and anxiety related problems and can interact with other CNS depressant drugs and CNS stimulant drugs.

For further information about drugs and their effects see DrugScope's website which has an 'A-Z of drugs' www.drugscope.org.uk/resources/drugsearch/drugsearch-index.htm

Commonly used drugs and their effects

Alcohol is by far the most popular drug in the UK. Hazardous and harmful drinking, and dependent drinking, is associated with a wide range of adverse health and social outcomes (SIGN 2003, HM Government 2007, Scottish Government 2009a). Alcohol is a CNS depressant drug which is easily absorbed into the bloodstream. It starts to take effect after approximately 5–10 minutes and its effects can last for several hours, depending on the amount consumed (DrugScope 2010). Its sedative effect slows the body down, making people feel relaxed and less inhibited. Higher consumption levels are associated with slurred speech, poor co-ordination, and drowsiness. Drinking too much can lead to loss of consciousness and death (normally by choking on vomit), and is associated with a higher risk of accidents, unprotected sex, aggression and violence (including domestic abuse). Tolerance to alcohol can develop with regular excessive drinking. Dependence is associated with withdrawal symptoms, which can be severe and lead to hospitalisation on account of confusion, hallucinations and seizures (commonly known as delirium tremens or the 'DTs'). Alcohol, taken in combination with other drugs such as opiates, benzodiazepines, and anti-depressants, is a common feature of fatal overdoses (DrugScope 2010).

Sensible drinking guidelines for men and women are far lower than most people think. The recommended guideline is that women should not regularly drink more than 2–3 units per day, and men should not regularly drink more than 3–4 units per day. Over the course of a week, women should not exceed 14 units and men should not exceed 21 units. In addition, guidelines recommend that everyone should have at least two alcohol free days per week, and should not binge drink (HM Government 2007, Scottish Government 2009a).

Please note: Guidelines on alcohol consumption for men and women trying to conceive, and for pregnant and breastfeeding women, are different. These are detailed in the next section of the resource book.

Benzodiazepine drugs, such as diazepam (Valium®), are commonly called 'minor tranquillisers' (anxiolytics) or 'sleeping tablets' (hypnotics) and are CNS depressant drugs. That is, they are sedative drugs which relieve anxiety and tension and can slow down people's reactions and make them feel calm, drowsy, lethargic and forgetful (DrugScope 2010). Effects begin after approximately 15 minutes and can last up to 4–8 hours without repeating the dose. Benzodiazepines are easily available on the black market and are in widespread use. People can become dependent on benzodiazepines in a very short period of time if they are used continuously. Withdrawal from benzodiazepines, particularly sudden withdrawal, can result in severe anxiety symptoms, insomnia, irritability, confusion, hallucinations and seizures (similar to alcohol dependency withdrawal symptoms). Many people find it difficult to stop taking benzodiazepines and may need a gradually reduced dosage to do so. With regular use, benzodiazepines can become ineffective as sleeping pills after 2 weeks and ineffective to alleviate anxiety after 4 months (DrugScope 2010). The temptation is to continually increase the dosage to obtain the same effect. Although dependent benzodiazepine use is common, benzodiazepines are only really effective as short term medicines. Research shows that fatal overdoses commonly include benzodiazepines taken in combination with other drugs, especially alcohol (DrugScope 2010).

Opioid drugs are CNS depressant drugs that have an analgesic ('painkiller') effect. They include:
- opiates... derived from the opium poppy e.g. morphine and codeine, and
- synthetic analogues... e.g. methadone ('meth'), diamorphine ('heroin'), dihydrocodeine (DF118 or 'difs'), buprenorphine (e.g. Subutex®, Temgesic® and Suboxone®), dipipanone (Diconal®), pethidine.

Opioids produce a range of physical effects apart from analgesia. They depress central nervous system activity, including reflex functions such as coughing, respiration and heart rate. They also depress bowel activity, resulting in constipation. At higher doses sedation results and the user becomes drowsy and contented. Excessive doses produce stupor and coma. Tolerance and physical dependence develops with regular continued use. The physiological effects of long-term opiate use are rarely serious in themselves. They include respiratory complaints, constipation and menstrual irregularity (DrugScope 2010).

Opioid *intoxication*... commonly referred to as being 'stoned' on opiate drugs after the person takes a dose which is above their tolerance level. An intoxicated person may be unresponsive, have pinpoint pupils, respiratory depression (shallow and infrequent breathing), a weak and rapid pulse, and they may appear pale and have cold extremities.

Opioid *overdose*... is life threatening. Immediate medical attention and treatment is required – normally naloxone (e.g. Narcan®) is administered to reverse the effects of overdose. A person who has taken an overdose will have blue lips and cold skin, will lose consciousness and not respond to stimuli, develop respiratory failure and die (sometimes through asphyxia after vomiting).

Opioid *withdrawal* in adults... abrupt withdrawal is rarely life-threatening and is considered much less dangerous than withdrawal from alcohol or benzodiazepines. Withdrawal symptoms develop in dependent opiate users normally 24–72 hours after their last dose. Symptoms can include: nausea, vomiting, diarrhoea, insomnia, muscle cramps, goose flesh, cold and clammy skin, dilated pupils, runny nose and eyes, abdominal pains, sweating, restlessness, irritability, as well as intense craving for the drug. Physical symptoms normally subside without treatment within 7 days. For opiate detoxification during pregnancy see section 'Management of substance use during pregnancy'.

Stimulant drugs (also called *psychostimulants*) are substances which induce short-term enhancements in either mental or physical function or both e.g. increased alertness, wakefulness, arousal, locomotion and stamina. Stimulant drugs are commonly referred to as 'uppers' because their effects tend to have an 'up' quality to them and they increase nervous system activity, whereas drugs which are CNS depressants are commonly called 'downers' (DrugScope 2010). Many stimulant drugs increase heart rate and blood pressure, and result in a loss of appetite and a diminished sense of the need for rest/sleep. With higher doses, users tend to feel confident and energetic, have fast flowing thoughts and ideas and can feel (and act) as if they have superior mental and physical powers (DrugScope 2010). Paradoxically, stimulant drugs can trigger anxiety as well as relieve it.

Most stimulant drugs (e.g. amphetamines, cocaine and crack) take effect very quickly (depending on route of administration) and are short-acting (wear off quickly). Regular use can lead to psychological dependence and increased tolerance, so more of the drug is needed to get the same effect. Users may be tempted to keep repeating the dose to avoid feelings of lethargy, fatigue, anxiety and depression. Heavy use is often associated with lack of sleep and food and lowered resistance to infections. Panic attacks, psychotic symptoms (including paranoia, delusions and hallucinations), and a feeling of being 'wired' may also feature. Some users experience severe mood swings and can become very irritable and aggressive. Symptoms normally resolve once the drug is eliminated from the body (DrugScope 2010).

Injecting drug use

Although many drug users report taking drugs by oral administration (swallowing, snorting, inhaling or smoking), injecting drug use is common. Drugs that can be easily prepared for injection include:

- diamorphine ('heroin')
- buprenorphine (Temgesic®, Subutex®)
- dipipanone (Diconal® – which includes cyclizine, an anti-nausea drug)
- cyclizine (Valoid®)
- amphetamines ('speed')
- cocaine.

Please note: Suboxone® (a buprenorphine/naloxone formulation) is normally prescribed in preference to Subutex® (buprenorphine) as a way of reducing the likelihood of users injecting this formulation.

Injecting drug use and sharing needles and syringes and other injecting paraphernalia (e.g. spoons, filters, water, cups etc) remains a major public health concern. Guidance on needle exchange or *Injecting Equipment Provision* (IEP) is now available for professionals and aims to promote single use only of injection equipment (e.g. needles and syringes) and injecting paraphernalia (Scottish Government 2010b). Messages about the risks associated with sharing injecting paraphernalia need to be continually emphasised by professionals as many drug users do not perceive themselves to be at risk of blood borne viruses (HIV, hepatitis C and hepatitis B) – see also section 'Management of substance use during pregnancy'.

It should also be noted that repeated snorting of drugs like cocaine and amphetamines damages the membranes which line the nose (DrugScope 2010). The sharing of snorting and inhaling paraphernalia ('straws') between users is associated with an increased risk of hepatitis C (Fischer *et al* 2008, Aaron *et al* 2008).

Drugs and their effects on the developing baby

All women should be given information on the effects of smoking, alcohol use and drug use during pregnancy. Ideally, information should be given well before conception so that the woman has an opportunity to modify her substance use before she becomes pregnant (see section on 'pre-conception care').

The general answer to a question like 'I took some X before I found out I was pregnant. Is it likely to harm the baby?' is most often 'no'. However, outcomes depend on the substance used, the amount taken, over what time period, how it was taken, at what stage in pregnancy, and many other factors such as diet, general health and social circumstances. One unfortunate aspect of over-emphasising the likelihood of adverse effects is that it may persuade some concerned women to inappropriately consider termination. Others may suddenly stop their dependent drug use (which could be dangerous to the fetus) or avoid engaging with professionals because of exaggerated concerns.

Drug use is associated with increased rates of obstetric and paediatric mortality and morbidity and can affect pregnancy in a number of ways. During the 1st trimester, when fetal organs are actually forming, teratogenic (malformation) effects are the main concern. This is a time when the woman may not even know she is pregnant. During the 2nd and 3rd trimester the main concern is about growth and functional development. Impaired placental function and fetal growth can result in a low birth weight baby. Illicit drug use and fluctuating consumption of substances can increase the risk of preterm labour and result in early delivery. The risk of Sudden Infant Death Syndrome is increased and Neonatal Abstinence Syndrome is common in babies born to women who are dependent on certain drugs. Children exposed to too much alcohol *in utero* can be born with Fetal Alcohol Syndrome or Fetal Alcohol Spectrum Disorder (RCOG 2006a, BMA 2007a).

Many women with alcohol and drug related problems feel worried and guilty about the effects of their substance use on the baby and may appear reluctant to discuss these issues as a result (Klee *et al* 2002). Professionals need to give parents licence to voice concerns, fears and questions that they are reluctant to bring up spontaneously. Very often parents will be relieved when a professional raises the subject and encourages them to share their concerns. Allowing them to voice anxieties about poor outcome and their ambivalence about their current situation, including their substance use, treatment and so on can be therapeutic. Parents often complain that they are not 'told enough' and professionals comment that parents are 'ill prepared' or 'ill informed'.

Service user information leaflets, such as the one included with this resource book 'Pregnant... and using alcohol or drugs?' (see appendix 4) should be given to all mothers who report problem substance use. This leaflet can be given to the woman when she discloses drug dependence or an alcohol related problem at the booking appointment. The leaflet is 'user friendly' and outlines the general effects associated with substance use during pregnancy, advice about how to manage substance use during pregnancy, information on breastfeeding, blood borne viruses and Neonatal Abstinence Syndrome (NAS). Women and their partners should be advised to read the leaflet and discuss it with the midwife or other health care professionals involved in their care.

Evidence base

With the exception of tobacco, it has been difficult to establish clear and reliable information about the effects of specific drugs on the developing fetus and baby. Much of the research is methodologically flawed and findings are inconsistent and contradictory (Hepburn 2004b). This is because well controlled studies are difficult to conduct and pregnancy outcome is multi-factorial (Kaltenbach 1994, Lester et al 2004, Schempf 2007). It is the result of a dynamic interplay of genetic factors, physical and psychological health, nutrition, social deprivation and other environmental influences, quality of health and social care, as well as the effects of tobacco, alcohol and drug use. These confounding factors (which are often not controlled for in studies) have made it difficult to establish cause-and-effect relationships. This is particularly true when relating specific intrauterine fetal drug exposure to long-term developmental outcomes in children (Hogan 1998, Frank et al 2001, ACMD 2003).

Drug and alcohol related problems are closely associated with poverty, unemployment, homelessness, violence, offending and imprisonment, poor physical and psychological health, social isolation, and poor uptake of health and social care. These other factors may therefore account for many of the findings reported in the research literature (Craig 2001). There is also a moral dimension to what purports to be objective scientific evidence. Reports of adverse effects are more likely to be published than research reporting no adverse effects, irrespective of the scientific validity of the research (Koren *et al* 1989, Frank *et al* 1993). The following information on specific drug effects should be read with these limitations in mind.

Effects of tobacco

The risks associated with maternal use of tobacco are particularly well established (NICE 2008a, 2010b). There are many harmful substances contained in cigarettes. Nicotine, carbon monoxide and cyanide are thought to have the greatest adverse effects, reducing blood flow and oxygen to the fetus (Johnstone 1998).

Smoking during pregnancy increases the risk of infant mortality by an estimated 40% (NICE 2010b), and maternal smoking during the first 12 weeks of pregnancy (until the end of the 1st trimester) is responsible for up to 25% of all low birth weight babies (Scottish Executive 2001). Smoking tobacco causes a reduction in birth weight greater than that from heroin and is a major risk factor in Sudden Infant Death Syndrome (Scottish Executive 2003). Moran *et al* (2009) point out that the potential direct pregnancy complications associated with tobacco are similar to those from cocaine – both are linked to intrauterine growth restriction, placental abruption, premature rupture of the membranes, and preterm delivery. Babies born to heavy smokers may also exhibit minor signs of withdrawal, including 'jitteriness' in the early postnatal period (Scottish Executive 2003).

Although there is no convincing evidence that smoking cigarettes causes congenital birth defects, many pregnancy and neonatal complications are associated with smoking (NICE 2008a, 2010b). These include:

- miscarriage
- ectopic pregnancies
- placenta praevia
- placental abruption
- preterm premature rupture of the membranes
- stillbirth
- preterm delivery
- intrauterine growth restriction (IUGR) or 'small for dates'
- low birth weight
- cleft lip and cleft palate
- reduction in breast milk production

- Sudden Infant Death Syndrome (SIDS or 'cot death').

Studies on long-tem effects suggest that children of smokers suffer more serious respiratory infections in childhood and adolescence (e.g. bronchitis and pneumonia), and are at greater risk of developing asthma and middle ear infections (NICE 2010b). *In-utero* exposure to smoke has also been associated with psychological problems in childhood (e.g. attention and hyperactivity problems, disruptive and negative behaviour) and may have an adverse effect on the child's educational performance (NICE 2010b).

Second-hand smoke ('passive smoking') appears to present similar risks to the fetus and baby as maternal smoking, particularly in relation to an increased risk of low birth weight, preterm delivery, SIDS, asthma, ear infections and respiratory infections (Martinez *et al* 1994, U.S. Department of Health and Human Services 2006).

A number of factors are clearly associated with smoking during pregnancy (NICE 2010b). Pregnant women who smoke are more likely to be younger, less well educated, work in non-professional or non-managerial jobs, live in social housing or rented accommodation, and are single or have a partner who smokes. The detrimental effect of health and social inequalities on maternal smoking during pregnancy has led to a more targeted approach to those most in need.

Effects of alcohol

A 'safe' level of alcohol use during pregnancy has not been established. At all points along the continuum from occasional light drinking to regular heavy drinking there is conflicting evidence as to the possibility of damaging effects on the fetus (Gray & Henderson 2006). It has been found that alcohol use during pregnancy may potentially affect fetal brain and central nervous system development at any gestation. Alcohol readily crosses the placenta and high maternal consumption is clearly associated with teratogenic effects i.e. abnormal development of the embryo and fetus (BMA 2007a).

A key methodological problem in research studies is that accurate measurement of alcohol consumption is inherently difficult and therefore findings are by nature unreliable. Most measurements of alcohol consumption rely on maternal self report which is often imprecise due to biases resulting from poor estimation, poor recollection and the social stigma associated with heavy drinking during pregnancy (Gray & Henderson 2006, RCM 2010).

Low to moderate consumption

In a review by NICE (2008a), they found no evidence of harm to the unborn baby associated with low levels of alcohol consumption (i.e. <1.5 units per day) although, because of a possible increased risk of miscarriage they recommended that pregnant women should avoid drinking alcohol during the 1st trimester if possible.

A systematic review (Henderson *et al* 2007a) found no convincing evidence of adverse effects associated with low to moderate alcohol consumption during pregnancy – defined as less than 1.5 units per day or 10 units per week. However, the evidence was not strong enough to rule out any risk. Evidence from two meta analyses on moderate drinking – defined as between 3–21 units per week (Polygenis *et al* 1998, Makarechian *et al* 1998), and an expert review of moderate drinking by the *National Institute on Alcohol Abuse and Alcoholism* (Gunzerath *et al* 2004) also suggest that moderate drinking is not associated with deficits in fetal growth or birth defects. Small for gestational age babies, miscarriage, stillbirth, and preterm delivery have all been associated with moderate to heavy maternal alcohol use but not consistently (Gray & Henderson 2006).

In addition to volume of alcohol consumed, the pattern, timing and duration of alcohol consumption during pregnancy appears to be important. Studies on the effects of binge drinking during pregnancy (i.e. consumption of 6 units or more on one occasion), have found no convincing evidence of adverse effects, except an increased risk of poor neurodevelopmental outcomes (Gray & Henderson 2006, Sayal *et al* 2009). Frequent high dose 'binge' drinking is considered a greater risk to the fetus than steady moderate drinking (Gray & Henderson 2006).

Heavy alcohol consumption

Heavy maternal drinking during pregnancy, especially that associated with alcohol dependence and severe alcohol problems, results in a small number of babies being born with *Fetal Alcohol Syndrome* (FAS). The prevalence of FAS in the UK is unknown, but prevalence studies worldwide suggest that FAS occurs in approximately 1:1000 births (BMA 2007a).

The term 'Fetal Alcohol Syndrome' was coined by Jones and Smith in 1973 to describe a cluster of clinical features seen in children born to alcohol dependent mothers in the United States.

Fetal Alcohol Syndrome is characterised by:
- Fetal growth restriction (with subsequent low birth weight, reduced head circumference and brain size).
- Failure to thrive (the child remains below the 10th centile).
- A cluster of characteristic facial abnormalities e.g. short palpebral fissures (eye openings), thin vermilion (upper lip), flattened midface and smooth philtrum (section between top lip and bottom of nose).
- Central nervous system damage resulting in permanent impairment of brain function, including intellectual and neurological abnormalities and developmental delay. Common problems include learning difficulties, attention deficits, poor social understanding, hyperactivity, impulsive behaviour, poor coordination and planning, poor muscle tone, working memory deficits, receptive language deficits, executive functioning deficits (e.g. difficulty in organising and poor cause-and-effect reasoning), and the inability to learn from the consequences of their behaviour. Around 25% of children with FAS have an IQ score below 70 (Streissguth et al 2004).

Diagnosis depends on confirmation of prenatal alcohol exposure, although there is no clear consensus as to what level of exposure is toxic (teratogenic). 'Heavy' maternal drinking is largely undefined in the literature. As a guide, the '4-Digit Diagnostic Code' ranking system (Astley 2004), distinguishes between levels of prenatal alcohol exposure as 'high risk' and 'some risk'. According to this system, high risk exposure is equivalent to a blood alcohol concentration (BAC) of 100 mg/dL or greater, consumed at least weekly in early pregnancy. The National Institute on Alcohol Abuse and Alcoholism also defines 'heavy alcohol use' as drinking over 6 units of alcohol in one episode on 5 or more days during a 30 day period (U.S. Department of Health and Human Services 2000).

Not all babies of women who drink heavily during pregnancy develop 'full blown' FAS, and considerable research has been undertaken to examine factors which contribute toward the development of FAS. Many other confounding factors appear to be important. These include general physical health, nutrition, hormonal interactions, mental health (especially stress levels), domestic abuse, age, parity, smoking and other drug use, as well as social deprivation (RCM 2010, BMA 2007a,

Abel 1998). It is now generally accepted that FAS is a complex multi-factorial disorder in which exposure to heavy alcohol consumption *in-utero* interacts with other environmental factors and genetic predisposition (Gray & Henderson 2006).

Other 'fetal alcohol effects' associated with heavy drinking have been described, including '*alcohol-related birth defects*' (ARBD) and '*alcohol-related neurodevelopmental disorder*' (ARND). These partial forms of the syndrome, which show some but not all of the features of FAS, comprise more subtle deficits identified on behavioural, cognitive, psychological and educational tests. These different effects have led to changes in terminology that have sparked considerable debate since the relationship between maternal alcohol consumption and the development of a range of disorders is not fully understood, and careful differential diagnosis is required (Abel 1998, BMA 2007).

Together, the cluster of effects is known as *Fetal Alcohol Spectrum Disorder* or 'FASD' (RCOG 2006). Incidence of FASD in Western countries is estimated to be around 9:1000 births (BMA 2007a). There is some evidence that FASD can occur with moderate levels of prenatal alcohol exposure, although this is not conclusive. Women most at risk of having a child with FAS or FASD are those living in poverty and social housing, women who smoke or use illicit drugs during pregnancy, older mothers, women with poor nutrition during pregnancy, and aboriginal women (BMA 2007a).

FAS and FASD are lifelong conditions that have a significant impact on the life of an individual and those around them (BMA 2007a). The neurological and cognitive deficits associated with FASD mean that affected children may experience problems due to difficulties in learning, judgement, planning and memory. These include mental health problems, disrupted school experience, criminal behaviour, imprisonment, inappropriate sexual behaviour, and alcohol and drug problems as adolescents and adults (Streissguth *et al* 2004).

Rates of FAS diagnoses are known to be poor (Elliott *et al* 2006, RCOG 2006). Characteristics of FAS or FASD may not be initially apparent at birth and may change over time as the child develops. Neurodevelopmental problems are usually assessed after infancy and tend to persist into adult life. Similarly, facial features of FAS become more apparent from around eight months of age but then tend to become less apparent in later childhood. The most accurate time period for a diagnosis is between three and twelve years of age (Gray & Henderson 2006).

Although there is a great deal of evidence to show that *paternal* alcohol problems affect child development and behaviour, few studies have investigated the effects of paternal alcohol consumption on the risk of Fetal Alcohol Syndrome (FAS) or Fetal Alcohol Spectrum Disorder (FASD). Some studies have investigated the link between *paternal* alcohol consumption on pregnancy outcomes, primarily birth weight, preterm delivery and miscarriage. The conclusion overall is that there is no evidence of a significant paternal contribution. However, no studies have focussed on neurodevelopmental outcomes (Gray & Henderson 2006).

Effects of drugs (illicit and prescribed)

As stated earlier, studies examining the effects of drugs in pregnancy are fraught with methodological difficulties and multiple confounding variables producing inconsistent and contradictory findings (Kaltenbach 1994, LaGasse *et al* 1999, Lester *et al* 2004). Reported drug effects on the fetus are broadly similar and largely non-specific to the type of drug used (Department of Health 2007a). Intrauterine growth restriction (IUGR) and preterm deliveries contribute to increased rates of low birth weight and increased perinatal mortality rates (Hepburn 2004b). These outcomes are multi-factorial and are also associated with socio-economic deprivation, poor maternal health, stress and smoking (Department of Health 2007a). Schempf and Strobino (2008) point out that studies which have controlled for antenatal care and associated social, psychosocial, behavioural and medical factors have found that the direct effects of illicit drug use on birth outcomes have not been significant.

Cannabis (e.g. marijuana or 'hash')

Despite its widespread use, information on the effects of cannabis in pregnancy is generally poor. A review of cannabis by the World Health Organisation (1997) concluded that there was no good evidence that cannabis itself has a direct effect on pregnancy or the developing baby. Fergusson *et al* (2002) found no association between maternal cannabis use during pregnancy and an increased risk of perinatal mortality or morbidity. In regard to effects on birth weight, a meta-analysis of studies which adjusted for smoking (English *et al* 1997), found inadequate evidence that cannabis use, at the amount typically consumed by pregnant women, causes a reduction in birth weight. However, cannabis is normally mixed together with tobacco and smoked in a 'joint'. Tobacco causes a reduction in birth weight, increased risk of sudden infant death syndrome (SIDS or 'cot death') and many other pregnancy complications.

Benzodiazepines (e.g. diazepam & temazepam)

There is no conclusive evidence that benzodiazepines cause congenital birth defects or other serious adverse effects on the developing fetus (Moran *et al* 2009). However, an increased risk of low birth weight and preterm delivery have been reported (Wikner *et al* 2007), and most studies have investigated low dose use, whereas many drug users report high dose intake. Whilst there have been some reports of facial abnormalities (i.e. cleft lip and palate) following high dose benzodiazepine use in early pregnancy (Dolovich *et al* 1998), these findings have not been reliably reproduced (Wikner *et al* 2007). Maternal use of benzodiazepines near term can also result in 'floppy baby syndrome', where the newborn baby is lethargic, has reduced muscle tone and respiratory depression (Day & George 2005).

Dependent benzodiazepine use by the mother is clearly associated with withdrawal symptoms in the newborn baby (Department of Health 2007a, American Academy of Pediatrics 1998). Neonatal Abstinence Syndrome can be more severe and prolonged with benzodiazepines and the onset of withdrawal symptoms can be delayed, secondary to maternal opiate use – see *'Neonatal Abstinence Syndrome'* section.

Opioids (e.g. heroin, methadone, dihydrocodeine, buprenorphine)

Good evidence on the effects of opioids is fairly limited and dated, particularly on the long-term effects on the child (Messinger *et al* 2004, Bell & Harvey-Dodds 2008, Hunt *et al* 2008). There is no convincing evidence that opioids cause congenital abnormalities or an increased risk of significant or permanent neurodevelopmental impairment (Johnstone 1998, Messinger *et al* 2004).

Opioids are associated with an increased risk of:
- low birth weight
- preterm labour and delivery
- intrauterine growth restriction (IUGR) or 'small for dates'
- Sudden Infant Death Syndrome ('SIDS' or 'cot death').

Greater risk of preterm delivery has been associated with illicit (street) drug use, injecting drug use, fetal withdrawal *in-utero*, poor diet, and poor maternal health. Almario *et al* (2009) found that pregnant women who supplemented their methadone prescription with two or more illicit drugs (including cocaine, alcohol, opiates and marijuana) were more likely to deliver preterm than when taking methadone alone. A meta-analysis (Hulse *et al* 1997) found that the risk of low birth weight is also increased if the woman uses heroin, or heroin and methadone, rather than methadone alone. However, other studies which have controlled for cigarette smoking, quality of antenatal care and other risk factors have found no association between opiate use and low birth weight or preterm delivery (Schempf 2007, Schempf & Strobino 2008). Maternal opiate use has been associated with an increased risk of cot death, even after controlling for the effects of cigarette smoking (Kandell *et al* 1993).

Case reports of opiate withdrawal during pregnancy have reported an increased risk of miscarriage in the 1st trimester and stillbirth and preterm labour in the 3rd trimester (Luty *et al* 2003). Sudden opiate withdrawal is therefore considered potentially unsafe for the fetus, although the risks of withdrawal have probably been exaggerated in the past and can be minimised by appropriate drug therapy for the mother (Johnstone 1998, Hepburn 2004b) – see *'Management of substance use during pregnancy'* section.

Neonatal Abstinence Syndrome (NAS) is well documented in babies born to mothers who are opiate dependent – see *'Neonatal Abstinence Syndrome'* section. Affected babies normally develop symptoms within 24–72 hours following birth. Symptoms vary in severity and can last from a few days to several months before they fully resolve (Lloyd & Mysersough 2006). Methadone (because of its longer half-life) is associated with later onset and more severe and prolonged withdrawal symptoms than either heroin or buprenorphine (Cairns 2001, Jones *et al* 2010, Kakko *et al* 2008). Heroin use however, is associated with poor maternal health, poor antenatal care, and a greater likelihood of poor pregnancy and infant outcomes.

Studies investigating long term developmental outcomes of children exposed to opiates *in utero*, report inconsistent and contradictory findings, reflecting the confounding variables that exist within these studies (Kaltenbach 1994). On balance however, most studies suggest that the care-giving environment plays a more important role on child development than drug exposure to opiates *in utero* (Ornoy *et al* 1996, Burns *et al* 1996, Messinger *et al* 2004, Topley *et al* 2007).

Cocaine and 'Crack'

Evidence on the effects of maternal cocaine use is fairly substantial but inconclusive. Adverse effects on the fetus have been largely reported in heavy crack/cocaine users, rather than with 'recreational' or occasional users (Hulse *et al* 1997b, Hepburn 2004a). Cocaine is a powerful vasoconstrictor, restricting blood flow and oxygen to the fetus. There is no good evidence that cocaine is teratogenic (Bauer *et al* 2005), or has a significant adverse effect on long term developmental outcomes for children (Frank *et al* 2001, Messinger *et al* 2004).

Cocaine/crack is associated with an increased risk of:
- placental abruption (where the placental lining separates from the uterus of the mother with associated haemorrhage and fetal hypoxia)
- intrauterine growth restriction
- low birth weight babies
- preterm delivery.

A meta-analysis (Addis *et al* 2001) on the effects of maternal cocaine use on pregnancy outcomes found that 'only the risk of placental abruption and premature rupture of membranes were statistically associated with cocaine use'. Bauer *et al* (2005) found that growth restriction was most evident in the larger, more mature infants, and that high dose cocaine use in the mother can result in the newborn showing signs of intoxication at birth – symptoms include: irritability, jitteriness, tremor, high-pitched cry, excessive suck, hypertonia, poor feeding and an abnormal sleep pattern (Bauer *et al* 2005). Neonatal Abstinence Syndrome (NAS) has not been reliably reported (Scottish Executive 2003).

A systematic review (Frank *et al* 2001) on developmental outcomes in children exposed to cocaine *in utero* found 'no convincing evidence of an association with developmental toxic effects that are different in severity, scope, or kind from the sequelae of multiple other risk factors'. Studies, including the largest matched cohort study to date (Messinger *et al* 2004), appear to suggest that environmental risks (especially the care-giving environment) is a better predictor of mental, psychomotor, behavioural and language development in children than *in-utero* cocaine exposure (Frank *et al* 2001, Brown *et al* 2004, Bauer *et al* 2005).

Amphetamines (e.g. methamphetamine, 'speed' or 'whizz')

There is no conclusive evidence that amphetamine use directly affects pregnancy outcomes (NSW Department of Health 2006). However, amphetamine sulphate is a powerful CNS stimulant and heavy users tend to have poor health (due to poor nutrition, weight loss, anaemia and mental health problems). Like cocaine, amphetamines cause vasoconstriction with associated adverse effects on placental function and fetal growth. Withdrawal symptoms in the newborn baby have not been reliably reported with amphetamine use, although like cocaine, intoxication effects have been described (American Academy of Pediatrics 1998).

More recent research on neonates born to methamphetamine users in the USA have reported adverse effects similar to those found with cocaine and tobacco, such as low birth weight and small for gestational age, suggesting a direct effect on fetal growth since they appear to be dose-related (Smith *et al* 2006). Subtle neurobehavioural effects in the neonate have also been associated with heavy methamphetamine use (Smith *et al* 2008). These include decreased arousal, increased lethargy, poor quality of movement and increased physiological stress when aroused. The neurotoxic effects of methamphetamine may be greater than cocaine because of its longer half-life (Moran *et al* 2009).

Ecstasy ('E' or MDMA)

There is no conclusive evidence that ecstasy use directly affects pregnancy outcomes or causes malformations, however information in the literature is scarce (NSW Department of Health 2006). Prenatal ecstasy use has been considered in recent research investigating the causes of gastroschisis (an abdominal wall defect in infants). A case-controlled study (Draper *et al* 2007) found 1st trimester use of vasoconstrictive recreational drugs (such as cocaine, amphetamines and ecstasy) was associated with an increased risk of gastroschisis. However, research on the characteristics of pregnant women who use ecstasy shows that they report a wide range of risk factors that may compromise pregnancy and infant outcomes, including smoking, heavy alcohol use, polydrug use, mental health problems and poor social circumstances (Ho *et al* 2001). Withdrawal symptoms in the newborn baby have not been reported with ecstasy use.

Hallucinogens (e.g. LSD – lysergic acid diethylamide or 'acid', and 'Magic Mushrooms')

There is little evidence regarding the effects of hallucinogens in pregnancy. Most research dates back to the 1970s when interest in the subject first arose because of concerns over case reports of teratogenic effects and a possible link with chromosomal abnormalities. There is no evidence of congenital malformations and no conclusive evidence of other increased risks in pregnancy (Aase *et al* 1970, McGlothlin *et al* 1970).

Solvents and volatile substances (e.g. 'glue' and butane gas)

There is little evidence regarding the effects of solvent and volatile substance use during pregnancy. However, inhaled solvents may reduce oxygen supply to the fetus and symptoms of withdrawal or intoxication have been reported in heavy users. A number of young people die each year from the effects of volatile substances (usually as a result of arrhythmia) and women who continue to use volatile substances in pregnancy run the risk of sudden death (Johnstone 1998).

Anti-depressants/psychotropic medication

The prevalence of mental health problems in people with alcohol and drug problems is high (Department of Health 2007a). Some may be prescribed psychotropic medication in conjunction with their alcohol and/or drug treatment. Evidence on the risks of neonatal problems and impaired infant development following exposure to psychotropic medication in pregnancy and breastfeeding is limited (NICE 2007a). Neonatal toxic symptoms and withdrawal symptoms following delivery by mothers who received psychotropic medication during pregnancy have been identified, and there are concerns regarding the long term effects of such medication on the neurological development of the infant (NICE 2007a). Certain drugs for the treatment of mental health problems (e.g. lithium, valproate, carbamazepine, lamotrigine and paroxetine) have been associated with teratogenic effects and all antidepressants carry the risk of withdrawal or toxicity in neonates. For further information on the effects of psychotropic medication during pregnancy see *Antenatal and postnatal mental health: clinical management and service guidance* (NICE 2007a).

Management of substance use during pregnancy

Many women who are not truly dependent on alcohol or drugs will stop spontaneously as soon as they know they are pregnant. This applies to approximately 20% of women who smoke cigarettes, and 34% of women who drink alcohol, and to many women who use cannabis and other drugs 'recreationally'. It also applies to some 'controlled' opiate and benzodiazepine users (Johnstone 1998). For most drug use (excluding opiates) the immediate goal would be one of abstinence, although in reality this may be difficult to achieve for many women. Much support and dependency counselling may need to be offered to help the woman work towards this goal.

In addition, research shows that women who have substance use problems are more likely to have substance-using partners (Effective Interventions Unit 2002). A woman's partner can exert a powerful influence over her substance use. It is very important therefore, to include the woman's partner in any treatment and care plan so that the most supportive environment can be created. Evidence suggests that women who engage in treatment with, rather than without, their partner, have better outcomes (Effective Interventions Unit 2002).

Smoking cessation

Ideally, all women should be advised to stop smoking, or given help to cut down, before they conceive. General practitioners, pharmacists, and practice nurses can refer to smoking cessation programmes and can advise about nicotine replacement therapy (NRT). General practitioners can also prescribe bupropion (Zyban®) to help with nicotine cravings, however women who are pregnant or breastfeeding should not use bupropion (NICE 2008a, NICE 2010b).

During pregnancy a proactive and personalised approach to smoking cessation is required. Smoking cessation advice given in the antenatal period has been shown to be effective and can result in significant gains in birth weight (NICE 2008a, NICE 2010b).

A proactive approach would include the following:

- At first contact, ask the pregnant women about her smoking status and provide information about the risks of smoking to the unborn child and the hazards of exposure to secondhand smoke.
- Emphasise the benefits of smoking cessation at any stage during pregnancy.
- Offer personalised information, advice and support on how to stop smoking.
- Encourage the woman to use NHS smoking cessation services and the NHS pregnancy smoking helpline.
- Provide details on when, where and how to access smoking cessation support services.
- Consider offering 1:1 support or visiting pregnant woman at home if it is difficult for them to attend specialist services.
- Ask about the smoking status of the father/partner and encourage them to stop smoking as well and to use NHS smoking cessation services.

Pregnant women who are strongly nicotine dependent and unable to quit unaided, can be offered **nicotine replacement therapy (NRT)** following discussion with a health care professional or as part of smoking cessation programme, which includes an assessment of motivation, counselling and support, and a discussion on the risks and benefits of NRT, which is now licensed for use during pregnancy and breastfeeding. Nicotine levels in the body whilst on NRT are typically lower than those present during heavy smoking and the many other toxins emitted by cigarette smoke, such as carbon monoxide are avoided. If a pregnant woman chooses to use nicotine patches, she should be advised to remove the patches before going to bed at night.

Women who are unable to stop smoking during pregnancy should be encouraged to reduce their consumption. Studies suggest that cutting down smoking can significantly reduce nicotine concentrations and can offer some measure of protection for the fetus, with a 50% reduction being associated with a 92g increase in birth weight (NICE 2008a).

Most areas now have smoking cessation support groups and practitioners who have a specific remit for smoking cessation during pregnancy. Contact your local GP surgery, local pharmacy, health visiting or midwifery service for further information. Information leaflets on smoking cessation are available for women and their partners and can be given out during pre-conception and antenatal consultations. The National Institute for Clinical Excellence (NICE) also has guidance on NRT in their 'Information for Patients' leaflet (www.nice.org.uk).

Many women with drug and alcohol problems smoke cigarettes and may find it difficult to stop smoking. It is easy to forget the risks associated with smoking during pregnancy when working with women who are using a whole variety of other drugs. Many women themselves are more concerned about the effects of other drugs, especially opiates. Professionals need to remind themselves that providing information on the risks of smoking is important if they are to convey a balanced and consistent message on the subject.

Alcohol consumption advice

In the UK, governmental advice about alcohol consumption during pregnancy adopts a precautionary approach and recommends that women avoid drinking alcohol when trying to conceive and when pregnant. The principle being that 'no alcohol is the safest option'. However, if women choose to drink alcohol during pregnancy, then the advice is to:

- drink no more than 1 to 2 units of alcohol once or twice a week,
- avoid alcohol in the first three months of pregnancy (because it may be associated with an increased risk of miscarriage),
- avoid binge drinking and intoxication (as this may be harmful to the baby) (NICE 2008a).

Although there is uncertainty about a safe level of alcohol consumption during pregnancy, there is no evidence of harm to the unborn child when low levels of alcohol are consumed (NICE 2008a). Women who are concerned about low levels of alcohol use can be reassured that 1–2 units, once or twice a week, is unlikely to do any harm (RCOG 2006).

Abstinence during pregnancy is recommended in several countries including the USA, Canada, Australia and France. Commentators point out that recommending abstinence goes beyond our current evidence base and may have its own adverse effects (Abel 1998), such as producing maternal anxiety and guilt which in turn may have a negative impact on subsequent child development (O'Connor 2002). It also stigmatises mothers whose drinking may not have harmed their child, and it may deter some women from attending antenatal care, or it may negatively affect the quality of the relationship the pregnant woman has with their midwife or obstetrician (ACOG 2008). The issue is a contentious one which has sparked considerable debate.

It is important to remember that women with serious alcohol problems need an environment where they are more, not less likely, to disclose their alcohol use and to talk about any difficulties they might have in cutting down. The approach to care should ensure that the woman is not made to feel guilty or to blame for her alcohol problem and feels supported by health and social care services.

Alcohol units – a rough guide

Most countries define standard 'drinks' but in the UK we refer to 'units'. A UK unit contains 10 ml (8g) of pure alcohol (ethanol). Since alcoholic drinks in the UK indicate both volume and strength – the concentration of 'alcohol by volume' (abv), a straightforward calculation can determine the number of units contained. For example, a 750 ml bottle of wine at a concentration of 12% abv contains 0.12 x 750 = 90 ml alcohol = 9 units. Or volume (750mls) x abv (12%) ÷ 1000 = 9 units.

However, it should be remembered that concentration of alcohol in different types of beer and wines varies greatly. In addition, the size of a 'glass' of wine in restaurants and bars varies enormously. Also, standard measures are only used in bars and restaurants but measures poured in the home are likely to be different, and usually much larger!

As a rough guide:

One 'unit' of alcohol is the equivalent to:
- one small (25ml) measure of spirits (40% abv).
- half a pint of normal strength beer or lager (4% abv).
- half a 175ml glass of average-strength wine (12% abv).

One small (125ml) glass of average strength (12% abv) wine contains 1.5 units.

A pint of beer (5% abv) contains 2.8 units.

A 275ml bottle of alcopops (5% abv) contains 1.4 units.

A 2 litre bottle of strong cider (7.5% abv) contains 15 units.

Drinks Calculators, which can be used to calculate the number of units in most alcoholic drinks, and **Unit Measuring Cups**, which can be used to measure the number of units in individual drinks are helpful and can be obtained from NHS Board Health Promotion Departments.

An online alcohol unit calculator is available on Drinkaware:
www.drinkaware.co.uk/

A list of alcohol units for a range of beverages is included in Annex 1 of the
SIGN (2003) Guideline 74 *'The management of harmful drinking and alcohol
dependence in primary care'*. www.sign.ac.uk

Alcohol screening

Routine antenatal care provides an opportunity to screen for hazardous and
harmful levels of drinking, to deliver brief interventions for reducing alcohol
consumption, and to refer for specialist treatment (RCOG 2006, ACOG 2008).
Asking about alcohol consumption is now part of routine history taking at the
booking appointment.

Research shows that alcohol screening questionnaires (such as T-ACE and TWEAK)
can significantly improve detection of at-risk drinking during pregnancy and are
easy and quick to administer in antenatal settings (Sokol *et al* 1989, Bradley *et al*
1998, Chang *et al* 1999, Chiodo *et al* 2009). For example, the T-ACE questionnaire
is a simple four-question test that takes about one minute to ask and will correctly
identify the majority (approximately 70%) of hazardous drinkers during pregnancy
(Russell *et al* 1994). Examples of alcohol screening questionnaires are included in
appendix 5.

Chang *et al* (2006) also investigated the use of alcohol screening tools to identify
at-risk drinking in expectant fathers. Paternal drinking can have a strong influence
on maternal drinking and fathers can play an important role in helping pregnant
women to stop drinking or to cut down their consumption (Alcohol and Pregnancy
Project 2009). Both T-ACE and AUDIT were found to predict problem drinking in
male partners of pregnant women who were themselves T-ACE positive, suggesting
that the use of T-ACE may be a practical way for healthcare practitioners (e.g.
midwives) to identify hazardous drinking in both pregnant women and expectant
fathers (Chang *et al* 2006). Tailored alcohol brief interventions and treatment can
then be offered to the couple.

Alcohol brief interventions

Most women (95%) either stop drinking or substantially reduce the amount of alcohol they consume once they know they are pregnant, or when they are given advice to do so (Gray & Henderson 2006, NHS Information Centre 2010). However, 'at risk' pregnant drinkers include not only women who know they are pregnant but also women who do not know they are pregnant. An unplanned pregnancy may not become apparent for several weeks after conception, by which time damage from maternal alcohol use may have already occurred. In the United Kingdom Millennium Cohort Study, 58% of mothers said their pregnancy was unplanned (Dex and Joshi 2005).

Although there is little evidence on the effectiveness of brief interventions in populations of at-risk pregnant drinkers (Heather *et al* 2006), there is substantial evidence that brief interventions, harm reduction advice, motivational interviewing and relapse prevention techniques are effective methods of reducing moderate levels of drinking in many other populations (SIGN 2003, Heather *et al* 2006).

Delivering an alcohol brief intervention is appropriate when a pregnant woman:
- reports drinking above recommended levels i.e. more than 1–2 units, once or twice a week.
- reports episodes of binge drinking i.e. 6 units or more on any one occasion.
- obtains a 'hazardous' drinking score using the T-ACE or TWEAK test.

Alcohol brief interventions typically include some or all of the following elements, based on an effective strategy known by the acronym 'FRAMES' (Babor & Higgins-Biddle 2001, Heather *et al* 2006, Kaner *et al* 2007). The aim of a brief intervention is to increase the woman's awareness of her alcohol use and its potential consequences, and to motivate the woman to reduce risky drinking.

FRAMES

Feedback	Provide the woman with personal **feedback** regarding her alcohol consumption and the risks associated with alcohol use during pregnancy. Feedback can include information about the score of a screening tool such as T-ACE or TWEAK.
Responsibility	Emphasise personal **responsibility** for change and the woman's freedom of choice.
Advice	Provide clear **advice** to reduce alcohol consumption and the benefits of reducing consumption, in a supportive rather than an authoritarian manner. Clarify what constitutes low risk alcohol use during pregnancy.
Menu	Offer a **menu** of different strategies to reduce alcohol consumption, providing options from which the woman can choose what seems most sensible to her.
Empathy	Be **empathetic**, reflective and understanding of the woman's circumstances and point of view. A warm and supportive practitioner style is most effective.
Self-efficacy	**Reinforce self-efficacy** – the woman's expectation that she can change her alcohol consumption. Encourage her to make a personal plan to reduce consumption.

For further information see *Alcohol Brief Interventions (ABI) Antenatal Pack* on NHS Health Scotland website: www.healthscotland.com/documents/4096.aspx

Women who drink heavily **before** conception are more likely to continue drinking heavily during pregnancy without intervention, and concurrent drug and alcohol use is associated with poorer outcomes (Department of Health 2007a). If alcohol dependence is established, referral to a specialist alcohol treatment service is advised. Brief interventions are not effective with people who are alcohol dependent (Heather *et al* 2006).

If alcohol dependence is suspected, consider the following interventions:

- Ask the woman to describe in more detail her pattern of drinking and alcohol consumption before conception and since conception.
- Complete a 'drink diary' (see appendix 6) by asking the woman to detail what she had to drink on each of the previous seven days.
- Ensure the woman's midwife, consultant obstetrician, GP, health visitor and other 'key workers' know about the woman's alcohol consumption (preferably with the woman's consent).
- Arrange an appointment for the woman to see the consultant obstetrician or GP.
- Refer to an alcohol service for specialist assessment and help (gently broach this subject with the woman and obtain consent before referral).

Alcohol dependence and detoxification

Pregnant women who are unable to reduce high levels of consumption should be fast tracked into an alcohol service for specialist assessment and help. Any referral will be dealt with promptly and the woman will be offered in-patient and/or out-patient care depending on her circumstances. Referrals should be made in writing, with the woman's consent.

Dependent alcohol use is such a serious risk to the fetus that detoxification should be considered at any gestation, and can be repeated if necessary. The aim is to reduce total fetal exposure to alcohol (Hepburn 2004b). Tolerance to alcohol normally develops at high levels of consumption, however tolerance may develop at lower levels of consumption in some women who are polydrug users, or those with compromised liver function.

Sudden cessation of heavy drinking is potentially dangerous to the mother (because of delirium tremens and seizures) and may cause fetal distress. Alcohol dependent pregnant women should be advised not to suddenly stop drinking but to consult their GP as soon as possible. Alcohol detoxification requires close monitoring of mother and fetus under specialist medical supervision that includes collaboration with an obstetrician and alcohol specialist and is normally conducted in an inpatient setting (Plant 2001).

Although there is a lack of evidence on the effectiveness of pharmacologic interventions in pregnant women enrolled in alcohol treatment programs in relation to maternal and infant outcomes (Smith *et al* 2009), medication to protect against the medical complication of withdrawal (normally benzodiazepines or chlordiazepoxide) is considered preferable to the risks associated with uncontrolled withdrawal or continued heavy drinking during pregnancy. Disulfiram (Antabuse®) however, is contraindicated for women who are pregnant or breastfeeding because of the potential risk of teratogenic effects. Women who conceive whilst taking this drug should receive counselling before deciding to continue with the pregnancy (Plant 2001).

Since the effects of alcohol are associated with dietary deficiencies, the importance of a balanced diet and vitamin supplementation should be discussed. Liver function tests, including prothrombin time should be measured.

Although there is little evidence on the effectiveness of psychological therapies for dependent drinkers who are pregnant (Lui *et al* 2009), alcohol detoxification should be part of a package of care that includes relapse prevention and psychosocial support (see 'postnatal care' section). For further information see Heather *et al* (2006) *A summary of the review of the effectiveness of treatment for alcohol problems*, London, National Treatment Agency. www.nta.nhs.uk

Assessing drug related problems

It is important to establish an accurate picture of a woman's drug use during pregnancy so that appropriate interventions and care can be offered.

An assessment of drug use during pregnancy may include:
- taking a detailed history of the woman's drug use
- asking the woman to complete a 'drug diary' (see appendix 6)
- assessing drug-related harm (e.g. the physical, psychological, social, legal, financial, lifestyle consequences of the woman's drug use)
- assessing the woman's aspirations and motivation to change
- toxicology screening (to test for recent drug use)
- assessment of withdrawal symptoms
- tolerance testing or supervised self-administration of methadone.

Professionals who are involved in the assessment or care of a woman with a drug related problem should:
- Discuss the woman's care with her general practitioner or other prescriber.
- Refer the woman to an appropriate drug service if she is not already attending one so that an assessment can be made.
- Seek advice from the woman's drug treatment specialist.

Please note: toxicology screening (drug testing) is used for clinical purposes in drug treatment programmes and should always be done with the woman's consent – see guidance document in appendix 7.

Management of problem drug use

The key aim of professionals should be to attract and retain women in health and social care services (Hepburn 2004a, Department of Health 2007a). Much of the skill in drug management lies in planning realistic and achievable goals with each individual woman (Johnstone 1998). Professionals need to be careful not to force their own ideals or 'agenda' on the woman. Many women already feel guilty and worried about the effects their drug use may be having on their unborn child. If women feel they are not meeting the perceived expectations of professionals they may under-report their drug use and conceal any difficulties they may be experiencing. Trying to persuade a woman to reduce or stop her drug use may simply alienate her, lead to relapse and a sense of failure, and result in non-attendance. Different treatment options need to be considered in the light of the woman's aspirations and particular social and psychological circumstances. Drug use may have been an integral part of the woman's life for many years. She may have had a previous pregnancy whilst using drugs with no apparent ill effects. This may be reinforced by drug-using friends who have also successfully delivered healthy babies.

Different drug treatment options to consider include:
- Safer drug use advice and education
- Needle exchange and safer injecting advice
- Substitute prescribing
- Stabilisation
- Slow reduction
- Detoxification.

All of the above can be incorporated into a recovery care plan.

Safer drug use

Injecting and unstable drug use during pregnancy is associated with increased risks for both mother and baby (Bell & Harvey-Dodds 2008). These risks include:
- sudden death through drug overdose
- transmission of blood borne viruses (including HIV, hepatitis C and hepatitis B)

- other complications associated with poor injecting practices and the contaminants contained in non-pharmaceutically prepared street drugs
- intoxication and withdrawal states
- preterm labour and delivery
- multiple social problems.

Reducing illicit, unstable and injecting drug use during pregnancy is therefore an important goal to work towards.

Pregnant women who are injecting drugs can be referred to needle exchange services for supplies of sterile injecting equipment and injecting paraphernalia, as well as specialist advice about safer injecting practices. Many pharmacies also offer an injecting equipment provision service.

Substitute prescribing

Methadone maintenance therapy (MMT) is the most effective and generally accepted treatment for opiate dependent pregnant women (Kandall *et al* 1999, WHO 2004), and is recommended by the Department of Health (2007a). Follow-up studies suggest that women who enter methadone treatment programmes during pregnancy have better outcomes in terms of their pregnancy, childbirth and infant development, irrespective of continued drug use (WHO 2004, Department of Health 2007a). Women attending treatment services usually have better antenatal care and better general health than drug-using women not in treatment, even if they are still using illicit drugs on top of their substitute prescription.

Methadone is normally taken orally in liquid form (methadone mixture 1mg/1ml). It is used to help people stabilise their drug intake and associated lifestyle. Methadone is slowly absorbed and long-acting so it offers stability of drug levels for both mother and fetus and significantly reduces the likelihood of intoxication and withdrawal states, which have been shown to have an adverse effect on the fetus (Bell & Harvey-Dodds 2008).

There is strong research evidence (WHO 2004, Department of Health 2007a) for the benefits of methadone maintenance treatment when given consistently, in adequate dosage, with adequate supervision and in the context of psychosocial support. Identified benefits according to the research literature (Ward *et al* 1998, WHO 2004, NTA 2004, NICE 2007) include:

- reduction of injecting behaviour
- reduction of the risk of viral transmission (HIV, hepatitis B & C)
- reduction of drug related deaths
- reduction of illicit drug use
- reduction of offending behaviour
- improved social functioning.

Dihydrocodeine (DF118) is another opiate drug that is prescribed and has been researched for its comparative effectiveness with methadone (Department of Health 2007a). Likewise, buprenorphine (an opiate partial agonist) is also prescribed for maintenance and for drug detoxification programmes. Both dihydrocodeine and buprenorphine have been used as substitute drug therapy in pregnancy (Wright & Walker 2001). There is evidence to suggest that babies born to mothers on buprenorphine may be at lower risk of Neonatal Abstinence Syndrome than with other opiates. In a recent trial conducted by the *National Institute on Drug Abuse* (Jones *et al* 2010), buprenorphine was found to be superior to methadone in relation to reduced withdrawal symptoms in newborns. Buprenorphine is an approved medication for treating opioid dependence, but less is known about its effects in pregnant women and their babies (Johnson *et al* 2003).

Substitute drug treatment for benzodiazepine dependency lacks evidence on its effectiveness and there are concerns that long term benzodiazepine use may cause harm in the form of cognitive impairment and mood disturbance. Many drug users however, continue to use benzodiazepines and many are prescribed diazepam (Valium®). The recommended maximum daily dose of diazepam is 30mg (Department of Health 2007a). Women who are prescribed benzodiazepines are normally advised to reduce to the lowest possible dose during pregnancy that avoids withdrawal symptoms and illicit use.

Community based drug services provide a range of treatment and care approaches. Many people with a drug dependency are prescribed substitute drugs. Pregnant women drug users are seen as high priority for drug services and are normally seen very quickly after referral.

Please note: Patients who are prescribed substitute drugs such as methadone must be made fully aware of the risks of their medication and of the importance of protecting children from accidental ingestion – see '*Keeping children safe from alcohol and drugs in the home*' leaflet, appendix 2. Prescribing and dispensing arrangements should also aim to reduce risks to children (Department of health 2007a).

Stabilisation

Pregnant women who are opiate dependent should not be required to make a commitment to reduce or come off their prescribed opiate drugs. The emphasis instead should be on support and engagement rather than enforced reduction or abstinence (Wright & Walker 2007). Stabilised drug use should be the first goal to work towards and may take some time to achieve. The aim is to minimise the risks to mother and baby, not only during pregnancy and the neonatal period, but ideally in the long term. Stable drug use, a stable lifestyle and abstaining from illicit (street) drug use are successful outcomes of treatment. If non-prescribed opiate use persists, the methadone dose may need to be increased in order to achieve stability and to help the woman abstain from street drug use (Department of Health 2007a).

Some studies show that plasma levels of methadone decrease with gestation, particularly in the 3rd trimester (Bell & Harvey-Dodds 2008). This may be due to the increased fluid space and a large tissue reservoir, as well as altered metabolism of the drug by the placenta and fetus. Lowering the dose to avoid complications may therefore be inappropriate as the woman may require an increase in methadone dose during gestation (Bell & Harvey-Dodds 2008). Splitting the dose can reduce peak-trough differences in blood concentrations and so minimise intoxication and withdrawal effects (Wittman & Segal 1991). Advise the woman to try dividing her daily dose in order to overcome the need for an increase (Department of Health 2007a). Conversely, in the immediate postnatal period, a reversal of these effects may lead to increased methadone plasma levels with intoxication effects, in which case, the dose may need to be reduced. It is important to warn the woman about this effect as it may have implications for the care and safety of the baby.

Reduction

Slow reduction in pregnancy is also an option but should be gradual, stepwise and tailored to the woman's response. Women commonly report that they wish to reduce their consumption of methadone during pregnancy in order to reduce the likelihood of Neonatal Abstinence Syndrome (NAS), although the relationship between methadone dose and severity of withdrawals has not been clearly established (Department of Health 2007a). It is important that the woman understands this.

If the woman is dependent on benzodiazepines as well as opiates, then she should be advised to try reducing benzodiazepines first (Department of Health 2007a). Diazepam (Valium®) is the drug of choice to prescribe, as it is longer acting than other benzodiazepines. Diazepam should be prescribed at no more than 30mg daily, reducing fortnightly-monthly in 2mg to 5mg decrements. Methadone can be reduced weekly or fortnightly in 2.5ml to 5ml decrements. Dihydrocodeine ('DF118') can also be prescribed at no more than 30mg tablets x 15 per day, reducing one tablet per week for 15 weeks. Women who are on buprenorphine when they become pregnant should be managed by a specialist drug service.

The woman's stability should be reassessed at each stage of the reduction before proceeding further. If the woman has not relapsed back into illicit drug use (this can be confirmed through toxicology screening) and wishes to continue the reduction, then proceed. If the reduction is commenced early in the 2nd trimester (i.e. 13 weeks) it may be possible to achieve abstinence before delivery. However, the desire to achieve abstinence should always be weighed up against the risk of relapse and its consequences.

Detoxification

Detoxification from opiate drugs may be considered at any gestation, however it is normally recommended during the 2nd trimester in order to avoid any risk of miscarriage in the 1st trimester and preterm labour in the 3rd trimester (Department of Health 2007a, Luty *et al* 2003). Opiate detoxification is rarely fatal for the mother and less serious than withdrawal from alcohol or benzodiazepines, but can be very unpleasant and the relapse rate is high. In one UK study of 101 pregnant women admitted for in-patient opioid withdrawal, only 42 completed the detoxification, only 24 of those were successfully followed up after discharge, of whom only one remained abstinent at the time of delivery (Luty *et al* 2003).

Rapid benzodiazepine detoxification should be avoided as this can lead to withdrawal seizures (fits) in the mother and fetal distress (Department of Health 2007a). Detoxification treatment should be similar to that of alcohol detoxification. Hospital or residential admission is necessary to supervise a gradual titrated detoxification and to monitor the fetus. If necessary, repeat detoxification treatment can be considered throughout the pregnancy. The aim is to reduce total exposure to the fetus (Hepburn 2004b). However, the impact of relapse on the woman's health and social circumstances should be considered against the potential benefits of achieving stability on a low dose substitute prescription.

Detoxification should be discussed and agreed with the woman's consultant obstetrician and drug specialist/prescriber beforehand and should be part of a comprehensive package of care that includes relapse prevention (see 'postnatal care' section). It is really important that the woman understands the risks associated with relapse (including overdose) and is certain that detoxification is the right option for her during pregnancy. As a guide, detoxification from opiates would be considered an appropriate option if there was good evidence that the woman was stable on a low dose of methadone (<60 mg/day) and had intensive aftercare support in place. Detoxification from opiates is normally offered as part of an in-patient programme over a 7–28 day period, and should not be confused with stabilisation or gradual dose reduction (NICE 2007).

Psychotropic medication management

The obstetric management of women with mental health problems and the neonatal management of infants exposed to antipsychotic medication during pregnancy and breastfeeding is outlined in *Antenatal and postnatal mental health: clinical management and service guidance* (NICE 2007a).

NICE (2007) recommendations include:
- Referral to a specialist perinatal mental health service.
- Before treatment decisions are made, healthcare professionals should discuss with the woman the risks associated with treating and not treating the mental health problem during pregnancy and the postnatal period.
- If considered necessary for the woman's mental state, psychotropic medication should be maintained at the minimum effective dose during pregnancy and switching to a drug with a lower risk profile for mother and baby should be considered.
- Consideration should be given to dose reduction and/or discontinuation two to four weeks before the expected date of delivery, with recommencement after delivery.
- Neonates exposed to psychotropic medication during pregnancy should be monitored for withdrawal symptoms following delivery.

A final word:

Over the years, much emphasis has been placed on pregnancy being a 'catalyst for change' or a 'window of opportunity' for women to either stop using drugs or to reduce their drug use and many pregnant women will tell professionals that this is what they want to do. In the UK, as in other areas throughout Europe, experience has shown that this has not generally proved to be the case (Baldacchino *et al* 2003, Wright & Walker 2007). Many women who try to reduce or come off drugs during pregnancy are not successful (Luty *et al* 2003). However, all attempts that pregnant women make to improve their health and social circumstances should be supported by professionals and be regarded as a successful outcome of care.

Neonatal Abstinence Syndrome (NAS)

A group of drug withdrawal symptoms referred to as Neonatal Abstinence Syndrome (NAS) can occur in infants born to mothers dependent on certain drugs. NAS occurs because, at birth, the infant is cut off from the maternal drug supply to which it has been exposed *in utero*.

The classes of drugs that are known to cause NAS include opioids, benzodiazepines, alcohol, and barbiturates. Classical symptoms of NAS have not been consistently reported with solvents, hallucinogens, cannabis and most stimulants, including cocaine and amphetamines (Scottish Executive 2003, American Academy of Paediatrics 1998).

NAS is the most commonly reported adverse effect of maternal drug use during pregnancy, and is well described in babies born to opiate-dependent women (American Academy of Paediatrics 1998).

It is important for professionals to know about neonatal withdrawals, so that mothers, fathers and other carers (e.g. kinship carers and foster carers) can be supported to attend to the baby's needs and to provide the right kind of supportive therapy to assist in the baby's recovery.

Signs and symptoms of NAS

NAS symptoms are generally non-specific to the class of drug and differ from drug withdrawal symptoms seen in adults (Oei and Lui 2007).

NAS is characterised by central nervous system irritability, gastro-intestinal dysfunction and autonomic hyperactivity. Symptoms vary greatly, but the majority of infants born to dependent mothers (55%-95%) will show some symptoms of NAS (American Academy of Paediatrics 1998).

Common signs and symptoms which have been reported in babies born to opiate and benzodiazepine dependent women, include the following:
- irritability (marked tremor, easily startled, increased reflexes and excessive crying)

- hyperactivity (excessive body movements, face scratching)
- hypertonicity (increased muscle tone and rigidity)
- a fairly continuous high-pitched cry
- inability to settle or sleep after feeds
- excessive sucking (including fist sucking)
- increased appetite
- poor feeding ability (hungry but difficulty in sucking, swallowing and successfully completing a feed)
- regurgitation and vomiting
- frequent loose stools or diarrhoea (which cause peri-anal excoriation)
- poor weight gain or weight loss
- repetitive sneezing, yawning, hiccoughs, nasal stuffiness
- tachypnoea (rapid shallow breathing)
- respiratory depression
- increased pulse and heart rate
- temperature instability, fever (>37.5 C), sweating and dehydration
- mottling (discolouration of skin)
- excoriation (skin abrasions) from excessive movement (usually seen around the buttocks, back of the head, shoulders, and heels)
- seizures (fits).

Seizures occur rarely (in approximately 5% of infants) and may manifest up to 30 days after birth (mean age of onset is 10 days).

The onset, duration and severity of NAS

The onset, duration and severity of NAS symptoms vary greatly and depend on many factors, including the:
- type of drugs used
- duration of mother's dependency
- timing and amount of the mother's last dose
- metabolism and elimination of the drug by the infant, as well as the
- gestational age of the infant.

Data on possible dose related effects of methadone are controversial and inconclusive (Department of Health 2007a, American Academy of Paediatrics 1998), with some studies showing a positive correlation between maternal methadone dose and the development or severity of NAS (e.g. Dashe *et al* 2002,

Dryden *et al* 2009), and other studies showing no correlation (e.g. Berghella *et al* 2003, Seligman *et al* 2010). In practice this means that NAS severity is difficult to predict, certainly on an individual basis. Some women on low doses will have babies who develop severe symptoms and some women on high doses will have babies with only mild symptoms. Little data exists on the dose related effects of maternal alcohol and benzodiazepine use.

Symptoms normally present within the first 24–72 hours of birth, in approximately 75% of cases. Withdrawal symptoms in the neonate can present later, last longer and be more severe with methadone and polydrug use (Wilbourne *et al* 2000, Dryden *et al* 2009). The onset, duration and severity of NAS associated with buprenorphine appears to be similar to or less than that observed following *in utero* exposure to methadone (Johnson *et al* 2003, Jones *et al* 2010), and unrelated to dose (Lejeune *et al* 2006).

The onset of benzodiazepine withdrawal in neonates can be delayed (due to slow metabolism in the neonate) presenting as late as 5–10 days of age, and duration of withdrawal symptoms can be more prolonged than with opiates (Coghlan *et al* 1999). The onset of alcohol withdrawal in neonates however, is normally more rapid, with symptoms sometimes presenting within the first 12 hours of birth. Heavy tobacco use in addition to opiate and polydrug use has been associated with increased severity of symptoms and delayed onset (Choo *et al* 2004). Neonatal symptoms associated with cocaine and amphetamine use are thought to be intoxication effects rather than withdrawals, and the short duration of symptoms due to the short half-life of those drugs (Oei and Lui 2007). In addition, all antidepressants carry the risk of withdrawal or toxicity in neonates (Isbister *et al* 2001, Sanz *et al* 2005). However, in most cases the effects are mild and self-limiting (NICE 2007a).

Acute symptoms of NAS may persist for several weeks and irritability can last for several months (particularly with benzodiazepines). Withdrawal symptoms in preterm infants tend to occur later than full-term infants and are generally milder (Doberczak *et al* 1991, Dysart *et al* 2007). This is thought to be due to a number of different factors, including: their reduced total drug exposure *in utero*, the developmental immaturity of their central nervous system, the different metabolism of preterm infants, and reduced ability to communicate the distress of withdrawal. One large cohort study, however, found no relationship between gestation and development of symptoms (Dryden *et al* 2009).

Some babies may present with symptoms of NAS with no reported history of maternal drug use. If NAS is suspected then the neonatal paediatrician can confirm the diagnosis by toxicology screening of the infant and will discuss the results sensitively with the parents.

Assessment of NAS

Assessment of the infant is done using a standardised tool or formal assessment score chart, as this provides a more objective measure of symptoms, and the best guide for making decisions about treatment and care (Lloyd & Myserscough 2006).

Assessment is normally carried out using either the 'Lipsitz tool' or a modified version of the Finnegan chart (see appendix 8), where numerical values are allocated on the basis of the presence and severity of various symptoms. The main dimensions that are measured include irritability symptoms (high-pitched cry, sleep pattern, body movements etc) and gastrointestinal symptoms (feeding pattern, weight, skin excoriation etc). A score is allocated to each symptom for each time period (e.g. 9am-1pm, 1pm-5pm, etc). Total scores for each time period are then calculated and trends in the severity of the baby's condition are monitored. Any drug treatment administered can also be recorded on the chart. This allows the medical staff to monitor the effectiveness of the drug treatment and to titrate the dose according to the infant's presenting symptoms, weaning the baby off gradually. All maternity staff should make themselves familiar with the current NAS score chart in use and be able to explain its use to parents.

Applying the NAS score chart to preterm infants (<37 weeks) can cause difficulties as symptoms such as high pitched cry, poor feeding and tachypnoea could be over scored, whilst other symptoms such as sleep pattern, muscle tone and fever could be underscored. Preterm infants tend to be cared for in hospital so staff should seek advice from the neonatal paediatrician (neonatologist).

Preparing parents for NAS

It is important to prepare parents for the possibility that their baby might develop withdrawal symptoms (even if they are dependent on very low doses of medication) and to communicate this information to them sensitively, using a non-judgemental approach.

Parents who have an infant with NAS experience the same range of emotions as any other parent of a newborn baby who is poorly. Anxiety, helplessness, fear and grief are commonly reported feelings. In addition they often feel guilty and 'to blame' for their baby's condition and will require considerable support, reassurance and encouragement. Caring for a baby with NAS can be very stressful and parents will require a lot of patience. Involving the parents in all the decisions and choices about their infant's care and keeping them fully informed of the baby's progress is important.

Ideally, parents will have been given clear and accurate information about NAS in the antenatal period so that they are well prepared. At booking, midwives should give all drug and alcohol dependent parents the information leaflet 'Caring for a baby with drug withdrawal symptoms' (see appendix 9). This leaflet outlines in 'user friendly' language, what parents can expect and how they can help. The woman and her partner should be given an opportunity to read the leaflet then discuss the care of the baby and any questions or anxieties that they may have with the midwife.

Management of neonatal withdrawal symptoms

There is considerable debate about how best to care for babies with withdrawal symptoms, since the evidence-base for effective management is weak (Osborn et al 2005a, 2005b). Practice varies in terms of inpatient or outpatient management, with both approaches having potential advantages (Kruschel 2007).

The focus of care aims to:
● foster the parent/infant bond
● ensure the safe adaptation of the baby to extra-uterine life
● detect any evidence of NAS symptoms and provide appropriate supportive therapy or treatment if required.

Unnecessarily prolonged hospitalisation or placement away from the parents should be avoided if at all possible in an effort to keep mother and baby together, to enable effective breastfeeding, to promote bonding and appropriate parent-infant interactions, and to foster good quality early parenting practices (Scottish Executive 2003).

All known drug and/or alcohol dependent women are normally asked to stay in hospital for a minimum of three days (72 hours) following delivery so that the neonate can be observed for signs and symptoms of NAS. Most babies with mild to moderate symptoms can be cared for in the postnatal ward, using supportive comfort measures. Staff in the postnatal ward need to show parents how to use the *NAS assessment score chart* (see appendix 8) and encourage them to get involved in their baby's care from the very beginning. Parents should be advised to keep a close eye on their baby and report any concerns to staff. It is important to ensure that the NAS assessment score chart is 'user-friendly' so that parents can understand the scoring system, can make use of it, and get involved in the care of their baby.

Pharmacological treatment may be required for some infants with acute symptoms, although the decision about whether or not to use medicine to aid the infant's recovery remains a clinical decision. A cohort study (Saiki *et al* 2010) comparing the management of infants with NAS on the postnatal ward compared to the neonatal unit found that the proportion of infants who needed treatment was lower if cared for on the postnatal ward and length of hospital stay, on average, was also shorter. None of the babies in both cohorts were readmitted within a 2 month period following discharge.

Please note: naloxone (an opiate antagonist) should not be used to reverse opioid induced respiratory depression in neonates as this will induce an abrupt opiate withdrawal crisis.

Supportive therapy for infants with NAS

The use of supportive therapy has been shown to reduce the effects of withdrawal in neonates and should be implemented as soon as possible following birth (French *et al* 1998). Parents should be encouraged to take a lead role in their infant's care and should be taught how to use supportive measures so that they can care for their baby appropriately. One-to-one 'hands on' guidance for mothers, fathers and other carers (e.g. kinship carers and foster carers) is often needed in order to build confidence in handling a potentially fractious and uncharacteristic baby. In hospital, mother and baby should stay in a single room in the postnatal ward or neonatal unit if possible, so that a suitable low stimuli environment can be created for the baby.

The kind of guidance on supportive therapy that is normally given to parents includes the following responses to a range of common symptoms:

Crying and irritability
- Ensure the baby is kept in a quiet room and has calm surroundings – no bright lights or loud sounds that might upset the baby and make them more irritable. The aim is to reduce sensory stimulation.
- Handle the baby gently and as little as possible – this will reduce the level of stimuli and disturbance and will keep the baby calmer.
- Use a dummy or pacifier ('soothers') for non-nutritive sucking (except when breastfeeding).
- If the baby has a lot of 'skin-to-skin' contact, the baby will cry less. Ask the mother and father to read the 'skin-to-skin' leaflet.
- Humming, gentle rocking, gentle baby massages and a deep relaxation bath can sometimes help.

Feeding problems
- Feed the baby in a quiet place with minimal disturbance.
- Feed the baby on demand – frequent small feeds are normally better.
- Allow time for resting in-between sucking.
- Burp the baby very gently each time they stop sucking and after the feed as infants often swallow air due to their uncoordinated and weak sucking reflex.
- Gently support the baby's cheeks and lower jaw to help improve their efforts to suck and swallow.
- If the baby has a lot of 'skin-to-skin' contact, the baby will feed better.
- Try giving the baby a very gentle tummy massage to help with abdominal discomfort.
- Keep a record of all the feeds the baby takes so that intake of calories can be calculated, along with weight gain.

Sleeping problems
- Provide the baby with a quiet room to sleep in, with minimal disturbance. Keep the room dim (no bright lights) and avoid patting or touching the baby too much.
- Ensure the baby has a clean dry nappy – check for nappy rash and apply hospital formula nappy rash cream or zinc cream if needed.
- Ensure the baby has clean bedding and clothes which are free from vomit. The smell of vomit may make the baby sick again, and vomit can irritate their delicate skin.
- Ensure the baby is not exposed to cigarette smoke.

- Avoid getting the baby too hot.
- Soft, gentle music, humming or gently rocking the baby may help them relax and sleep.

Excessive movement problems
- Swaddle the baby (by snugly wrapping the baby up in a light soft flannel blanket with arms and knees bent into a comfortable position) – this may help with tremors, jerks and restlessness. A cotton baby sling can also be used.
- Keep the baby in a quiet room.
- Use soft flannel blankets or a short-haired sheep skin covered by a cotton sheet in the cot for the baby's comfort.
- Avoid handling the baby too much if it is very restless, jittery or trembling – keep any stimulation down to a minimum to help calm the baby.

Skin problems
- Regularly check and change the baby's nappy.
- Change the baby's clothes frequently, especially if they sweat a lot.
- Cover the baby's hands with gloves or mittens to prevent skin damage from too much fist sucking.
- Keep any areas of damaged skin clean – avoid baby lotions as the baby may suck them.
- To help prevent nappy rash and sores, apply hospital formula nappy rash cream or zinc cream around the baby's bottom area.

Breathing problems
- Ensure the baby is not exposed to cigarette smoke. The air should be clean and the room warm.
- Keep the baby's nose and mouth clean.
- Feed the baby slowly, allowing rest periods in-between sucking.
- Avoid overdressing or wrapping the baby too tightly.
- Keep the baby in a well supported semi-sitting position, and avoid putting the baby on its tummy to sleep.
- Advise the parents to keep a close eye on the baby and if breathing difficulties continue or worsen, contact the GP, midwife or health visitor, or dial 999.

Temperature problems
- Keep clothing to a minimum and avoid a lot of bedclothes – avoid getting the baby too hot.
- If the baby has a lot of 'skin-to-skin' contact, this will help to control the baby's body temperature.
- Advise parents to seek medical help if the baby has a high temperature for more than 4 hours. Call the midwife, health visitor or GP in the first instance.

Other problems
- Advise parents that if the baby has severe vomiting or diarrhoea and becomes dehydrated, to contact the midwife, health visitor, GP, or hospital for advice immediately.
- Likewise, if the baby has a convulsion (seizure), the parents should dial 999 and ask for an ambulance to take the baby to hospital.

Care in the community

After 72 hours stay on the postnatal ward, babies with mild to moderate symptoms can be discharged home where they can be cared for by their parents with support from the community midwifery, health visitor and other parenting services. The midwife will offer advice and support on a daily basis and will arrange for readmission to hospital if the baby's symptoms worsen. As part of the infant's ongoing care, parents should be advised to continue using the NAS assessment score chart for at least a week (until the baby is 10 days old). Supportive therapy measures should continue until the baby's symptoms have resolved. Parents should be advised to record all feeds (amounts taken and times) so that the midwife and health visitor can monitor the baby's daily calorie intake. The community midwife and health visitor will also weigh the baby to ensure weight gain is satisfactory.

If the baby's symptoms get significantly worse at home (i.e. sleeps less than 1 hour/cries 1 hour after feeds/weight loss after day 7) then admission to hospital should be considered. If the baby has been home for less than a week, or is less than 10 days old they may be admitted to the Neonatal Unit. If the baby is more than 10 days old they are normally admitted to the Children's Hospital.

Care in hospital

Parents need to know that admission to the Neonatal Unit or SCBU may be necessary if their baby develops severe withdrawal symptoms. Babies with severe symptoms sometimes require 'tube' feeding, pharmacological (drug) treatment and 24-hour care and supervision from specialist paediatric medical and nursing staff. Involvement of the parents in the care of the baby however, is still crucial to the infant's recovery.

The aim of treatment in the neonatal unit is to:
● reduce irritability and motor instability
● establish an appropriate feed/sleep/wake cycle
● maintain a normal body temperature, and
● ensure adequate weight gain.

Babies with severe symptoms usually stay in the neonatal unit for about 10 days (Dryden *et al* 2009), but sometimes for much longer (Lloyd & Myserscough 2006). Mothers are encouraged to 'board' (rooms permitting) in the hospital whilst their baby is in the unit (particularly if they are breastfeeding) or at least have substantial daily contact to continue the bonding process.

The use of pharmacological management for babies affected by NAS can reduce duration and severity of symptoms, compared to supportive therapy measures (Osborn *et al* 2005a, 2005b), although few studies have evaluated the benefits of different treatment agents and strategies (Kruschel 2007). Practice varies from unit to unit, with some neonatal units treating a large percentage of affected babies, whilst other units not opting for pharmacological treatment unless absolutely necessary – for example, to treat babies who have seizures. Drug management is decided by the attending physician but normally includes the use of one or more of the following drugs: oral morphine, diazepam, phenobarbitone, clonidine, and chlorpromazine. The best drug appears to be morphine if the main drug used by the mother has been an opioid (Osborn 2005a, 2005b, Ebner *et al* 2007). More recently, buprenorphine has also been used to treat infants (Kraft *et al* 2008). Where other drugs (e.g. benzodiazepines) have been used alone or in combination, drug therapy may need to be individually tailored towards a longer or biphasic pattern of withdrawal (Shaw 1999). Care is taken not to sedate the baby and to wean them off medication as soon as possible. Babies can be discharged home as soon as they are well enough to be cared for by their parents.

Blood borne viruses and pregnancy

HIV, hepatitis B and hepatitis C are all blood borne viruses (BBVs) that can be passed from mother-to-child (vertical transmission).

All professionals have a role to play in:
- Raising awareness of blood borne viruses
- Providing advice about how to reduce the risk of transmission
- Promoting testing
- Enabling people to attend treatment and care services.

Antenatal testing for HIV, hepatitis B, hepatitis C

In the UK, testing for HIV and hepatitis B (HBV) is recommended as part of routine antenatal screening. The aim of testing women during pregnancy is to reduce the likelihood of mother-to-child transmission, and to improve and protect the health of both mother and baby. Testing for hepatitis C (HCV) should be offered to those at risk, but is *not* part of the routine antenatal screening programme (RCM 2008b). The aim of testing is to identify infected women and to allow testing of their children so that mother and child/ren can be offered treatment if required.

All pregnant women receive detailed written information about routine antenatal screening tests. At the booking appointment the midwife will ask the pregnant woman whether she has read and understood the leaflet. The benefits and risks of each test, and their implications are discussed briefly before informed consent is obtained and blood is taken. All tests are carried out unless the women specifically requests otherwise. Women can 'opt out' of any test, if they wish. Testing for hepatitis C with women at risk during pregnancy requires specific discussion and informed consent (RCM 2008b).

All negative results should be communicated to the woman at her next antenatal appointment and are recorded in the woman's maternity records.

If an HIV antibody, hepatitis C PCR (RNA viral load), or hepatitis B (HBsAg) test is positive the virologist should report the results to the designated lead obstetrician and/or specialist midwife responsible for blood borne viruses. The obstetrician/

midwife recalls the woman so that she can be given the results in person, and blood can be taken to confirm the result. At this visit, support, treatment and care are discussed and issues of confidentiality and disclosure are addressed. In addition, there is appropriate referral to specialist teams for blood borne viruses.

The Royal College of Obstetricians and Gynaecologists (RCOG 2010) provides further **good practice guidance** on antenatal HIV testing, including:

- If a pregnant women declines an HIV test, this should be documented in the woman's maternity notes, her reasons should be sensitively explored, and screening should be re-offered again at around 28 weeks gestation.
- If a woman tests HIV negative at booking, but is judged to be at continued high risk of acquiring HIV, a repeat HIV test should be considered.
- Where a woman books for antenatal care at 26 weeks gestation or later, the HIV test should be requested urgently and the result issued within 24 hours.
- Rapid HIV test devices, which can deliver results within 20 minutes of the sample being taken, should be offered to all pregnant women whose HIV status in labour is unknown. A reactive result should be acted upon immediately.

If a woman refuses an HIV test, both antenatally and when in labour, an HIV test may be considered for the infant – see UK National Guidelines for HIV Testing (BHIVA *et al* 2008).

HIV (Human Immunodeficiency Virus)

HIV is the virus that causes AIDS (Acquired Immune Deficiency Syndrome). HIV can be passed from mother to baby during pregnancy (intrauterine), childbirth (intrapartum) and through breastfeeding. The risk of transmission is related to maternal health, obstetric factors and infant prematurity (BHIVA/CHIVA 2008). The majority of vertical transmission (around 80%) occurs during the intrapartum period and there is a close correlation between maternal viral load and risk of transmission – the higher the viral load the greater risk of transmission. Breastfeeding is also an important route of transmission. The additional risk of transmission through breastfeeding, over and above the intrauterine and intrapartum contribution, is estimated to be between 14% and 28% (RCOG 2010).

Without treatment, the mother-to-baby transmission rate is approximately 15%-25%. With no treatment, HIV-infected children develop chronic disease and about 20% develop AIDS or die in the first year of life. By the age of 6 years, about 25%

will have died and most surviving children will have some illness because of their infection. The long-term picture is unknown, but all children with HIV benefit from early life-prolonging treatment (BHIVA/CHIVA 2008).

The aim of the antenatal screening programme is to reduce the number of babies born with HIV and to improve the health of infected women and their babies. Diagnosis in pregnancy means that women can be offered advice, treatment and interventions to reduce the likelihood of mother-to-baby transmission. If appropriate interventions are accepted, the risk of vertical transmission can be reduced to less than 2% (BHIVA/CHIVA 2008).

Recommended interventions to prevent mother-to-child transmission are set out in the British HIV Association (BHIVA) and Children's HIV Association (CHIVA) *Guidelines for the management of HIV infection in pregnant women* (De Ruiter *et al* 2008), and the Royal College of Obstetricians and Gynaecologists *Green-top Guideline no.39: Management of HIV in Pregnancy* (RCOG 2010).

Interventions include:
- The use of antiretroviral drugs for both mother and baby
- Careful obstetric management during pregnancy and delivery
- Delivery by pre-labour caesarean section, where indicated
- Avoidance of breastfeeding.

The full BHIVA/CHIVA guidelines (De Ruiter *et al* 2008), with an appendix on safety and toxicity data is available on the BHIVA website: www.bhiva.org

Management of HIV positive pregnant women and their babies

The care offered to HIV positive pregnant women and their babies is jointly managed by a multi-disciplinary team including Midwifery, Obstetrics, HIV Specialists, Paediatrics, Primary Care and other services e.g. pharmacists, drug services and social work where appropriate. Healthcare staff should refer to their agreed management protocol and care pathway. The approach to treatment is individualised, according to the needs and choices of each mother. Good liaison is required between all professionals to ensure that the pregnancy and birth plan proceed appropriately and that the views and wishes of the woman are respected.

There are two scenarios in which HIV infection may be identified during pregnancy:
1. through antenatal testing, or

2. when a woman discloses her known positive status when booking.

Women who are newly diagnosed HIV positive should have an early assessment of their social circumstances, and all women should be encouraged to disclose their HIV status to their partner and given appropriate support (RCOG 2010). Care should be taken to avoid inadvertent disclosure of the woman's positive status to family members and friends – for example, even if they attend antenatal or postnatal appointments or are present at the delivery (RCOG 2010). In the context of multi-agency working, a positive HIV diagnosis should only be disclosed on a 'need to know' basis, and must be handled discreetly and sensitively.

All professionals supporting HIV infected pregnant women should be aware of the psychosocial issues that can impact on HIV treatment and care (BHIVA/CHIVA 2008). Women may need considerable help and support to come to terms with the implications of their diagnosis and the management of their infection. Guidance and support for woman should take into account their personal circumstances as well as any specific social or cultural issues. This may include fear of domestic abuse, relationship breakdown or rejection from family and friends.

Antiretroviral drug therapy (ART) for the mother aims to reduce her viral load to 'undetectable' (<50 copies/ml). ART is given according to the mother's HIV health status. For women who **do not** need HIV treatment for their own health, treatment is normally deferred until just before the 3rd trimester (around 20–28 weeks) in order to reduce fetal exposure, and the mother stops taking ART after the baby is delivered. For women who **do** require HIV treatment for their own health, ART is normally prescribed throughout pregnancy and postpartum. The goal in both scenarios is to maintain the woman's viral load to below 50 copies/ml.

The recommended **mode of delivery** is also dependent on viral load. Caesarean section is recommended if the viral load result is >1000 (>50 copies/ml). If the viral load is <1000 (ideally <50 copies/ml) at term then vaginal delivery is considered an acceptable choice for the mother (De Ruiter *et al* 2008). A decision about mode of delivery should be made at 36 weeks after discussion with the woman (RCOG 2010).

Vaginal delivery is accompanied by careful monitoring and obstetric management, such as:
● Shortened labour
● No instrumental delivery

- No artificial rupture of membranes
- No invasive procedures such as fetal blood sampling and fetal scalp electrodes
- No episiotomy.

There should be strict criteria for induction of labour and also for augmentation or acceleration of labour. In the event of any delays, there will be an accumulated risk of having to proceed to a Caesarean section. A copy of the woman's *care plan* should be kept in the maternity unit, labour suite and neonatal unit. This should include a summary of the treatment required during labour and the medication and follow-up required for the baby. The woman herself should also carry a copy of her care plan and present to labour ward on admission. This is particularly useful in the event of unavoidable admission to another maternity hospital that does not have her records or an appropriate protocol in place.

The Royal College of Obstetricians and Gynaecologists (2010), recommends that **HIV positive women should be advised not to breastfeed.** The risk of transmission through breastfeeding even when the mother has an undetectable viral load is uncertain (RCOG 2010). Maternal viral load is known to be a poor marker of the HIV virus level in breast milk, and although ART is likely to reduce free virus in the plasma and cell-associated virus in breast milk, the presence of HIV DNA remains unaffected and may therefore, pose a transmission risk (De Ruiter *et al* 2008). Consequently, advice to HIV positive mothers living in the UK, where safe infant feeding alternatives are available and free for women in need, is to feed their baby exclusively with artificial (formula) milk.

Infant feeding support for HIV positive mothers (RCOG 2010), should include the following:

- Support and advice on infant formula feeding – this is especially important for women whose families are unaware of their HIV status and where the cultural norm is to breastfeed
- Medication to suppress breast milk production (given within 24 hours of delivery).
- Guidance about the importance of contraception when not breastfeeding.

Antiretroviral drug therapy (ART) is normally given to the **baby** for the first 4 weeks. The lead paediatrician for BBVs determines the choice of ART. Medication for the infant should be given as soon as possible after birth (no more than four hours) and the administration times strictly adhered to (RCOG 2010). Infants born preterm are at most risk of HIV infection and are more difficult to treat. Detailed guidance on ART for infants is included in the BHIVA/CHIVA guidelines (De Ruiter *et al* 2008).

The lead paediatrician undertakes **diagnosis of HIV infection in infants** born to HIV positive mothers. All babies born to mothers infected with HIV will test HIV-antibody positive at birth due to the presence of maternal HIV antibodies. Babies who are not infected will become HIV antibody negative by 18 months of age. Other tests (using PCR techniques which test for HIV DNA) are used to diagnose infants before the age of 3 months. Infants are therefore tested at day 1, 6 weeks and 12 weeks of age. If all these tests are negative and the baby is not being breastfed, the parents can be informed that the child is not HIV-infected (De Ruiter *et al* 2008). A confirmatory HIV antibody test is performed at around 18 months of age.

Most neonates born to mothers known to have HIV will be exposed to ART *in utero*. The possible adverse effects of ART to the fetus and developing child are closely monitored, and a named paediatrician is normally responsible for the follow-up of all babies born to HIV positive mothers within a designated area. To date, no increased risk of birth defects, or growth and developmental problems, have been documented with zidovudine (ZDV) monotherapy – previously known as AZT. However, much less is known about the long term safety of other antiretroviral drugs (De Ruiter *et al* 2008).

All HIV positive pregnancies, all infants born to HIV infected women, and all children with HIV infection (including those who were born abroad and came to the UK and Ireland later) are registered anonymously with the *National Study of HIV in Pregnancy and Childhood* – see details at www.nshpc.ucl.ac.uk. In addition, all pregnant women taking ART are registered with the Antiretroviral Pregnancy Register www.apregistry.com, and all infants exposed to ART are registered with the British Paediatric Surveillance Unit www.bpsu.inopsu.com.

HIV prevention and child welfare issues

In rare cases, women may not accept recommended interventions to reduce the risk of mother-to-child transmission. For example, a woman may:

- refuse ART treatment for herself
- refuse to undergo a Caesarean section where indicated
- decide to breastfeed against clear advice not to do so
- refuse ART treatment for the baby
- decline HIV testing for the infant, and perhaps her other children.

Common reasons for this include: difficulty in coming to terms with the HIV diagnosis, religious reasons, fear of disclosure to partners, stigma, and other family members advising the woman against accepting the recommended interventions (De Ruiter *et al* 2008).

Where a woman refuses interventions to reduce the risk of mother-to-child transmission, despite all efforts by the multidisciplinary team to influence her decision-making, a pre-birth planning meeting should be held with social services to discuss child welfare issues (RCOG 2010). This meeting should provide a co-ordinated approach to explore the complexities of the situation with the parents so that they fully understand the potential implications of their decisions. The parents should be informed that it is the paediatrician's role to advocate on behalf of the child's wellbeing and to prevent, where possible, HIV infection (De Ruiter *et al* 2008). This may involve preparation of a legal case to treat the infant with ART, prevent breastfeeding, test the infant for infection, and ensure the infant attends for follow-up care, irrespective of the parents' wishes.

HIV positive parents with existing children of unknown HIV status should be encouraged to have the children tested. Lack of symptoms does not mean HIV negativity, even in teenage children (De Ruiter *et al* 2008). Detailed guidance about HIV testing of children whose parents are known to be HIV positive is available from BHIVA www.bhiva.org/DontForgettheChildren.aspx and is included in the BHIVA, BASHH, BIS (2008) publication *UK National Guidelines for HIV Testing 2008* – see Appendix 5: Testing of infants, children and young people.

Hepatitis B (HBV)

Hepatitis B is a virus which affects the liver and is highly infectious. It can be passed from mother-to-baby during childbirth – approximately 80–90% transmission rate from infectious 'carrier' mothers. There is no evidence to suggest that the risk of hepatitis B infection is increased through breastfeeding, so breastfeeding can be promoted (WHO 1996).

People who remain chronically infected with hepatitis B (i.e. 'carriers') can remain well for many years and may not know they are infected. Babies who are infected – and who become a chronic carrier (up to 90%) – are at risk of developing serious liver disease later in life.

Preventing HBV infection

Treatment to reduce the risk of transmission from mother-to-baby is now recommended for mothers with a high viral load (around 200,000 IU and above). An oral antiviral tablet (tenofovir) can be safely administered during the last trimester of pregnancy, normally 28 weeks to term (Tran 2009).

The high rate of mother-to-baby transmission can also be largely prevented through **immunisation**. If the antenatal hepatitis B surface antigen test is positive, a vaccination programme is started at birth to enable the baby to develop immunity and to have a healthy life. The midwife delivering intrapartum care should notify the neonatal paediatrician that the woman is in labour and ensure that the medications for the baby are in stock. Within 12 hours of birth the baby must be given the first hepatitis B vaccine dose. Babies who are at high risk of transmission are also given hepatitis B specific immunoglobulin at the same time (immunoglobulin neutralises the virus) (Salisbury *et al* 2006). The second dose of vaccine is given at one month, third dose at two months and fourth dose at twelve months. Infection and immunity checks are carried out at 15–18 months of age. The GP and health visitor must be informed, as they are responsible for ensuring that the baby receives all the vaccines to complete the immunisation programme.

It is important to trace any potential contacts e.g. sexual partners, children and other household contacts, so that they can be offered testing and immunisation if non-immune. Newly diagnosed mothers should also be referred to the Liver Specialist or Infectious Diseases Unit for assessment and follow-up.

Drug use and hepatitis B

It is **good practice** to offer all women with a history of injecting drug use (or a sexual partner with a history of drug use) full screening for HBV in pregnancy (i.e. the *Ab* test in addition to the *Ag* test). Women with no prior infection with HBV (non-immune) can be safely immunised during pregnancy (RCOG 2010). Current sexual partners, other household members, and existing children should also be immunised. Hepatitis B and hepatitis A immunisation is recommended for any hepatitis C positive or HIV positive woman (BHIVA/CHIVA 2008).

General practitioners, midwives, health visitors and drug workers are all in a good position to raise the subject of hepatitis B, and to recommend screening and immunisation. Immunisation can now be easily carried out in general practice.

Hepatitis C (HCV)

Hepatitis C is a virus which affects the liver and can be passed from mother to baby, either during pregnancy or childbirth, but not through breast feeding. People who are chronically infected with hepatitis C can remain well for many years and may not know they are infected. Babies who are infected through vertical transmission are at increased risk of developing serious liver disease later in life. There is a slow, non-linear progression of fibrosis with age, and the mean time to development of cirrhosis is estimated at 28 years (SIGN 2006). Some infected children will develop severe hepatitis or cirrhosis in childhood, although this is rare (<5%).

Pregnant women who are HCV antibody positive and HCV RNA negative (i.e. not chronically infected) do not pose a risk of transmission to their child (SIGN 2006). Mother-to-child transmission can only occur when the pregnant women is HCV antibody positive and HCV RNA positive (i.e. is chronically infected). The transmission rate is low (<6%).

Unfortunately, there is no vaccine currently available to prevent hepatitis C infection. Combination therapy drug treatment for hepatitis C (interferon & ribavirin) is contraindicated during pregnancy and breastfeeding (because of the fetotoxic and teratogenic effects of ribavirin) and in young infants. As yet, there are no proven interventions to prevent or reduce the risk of vertical transmission (except in the case of co-infection, see below). **Breastfeeding can be encouraged** as there is no evidence that HCV can be transmitted by this route (SIGN 2006). Universal screening of all pregnant women is therefore not currently recommended. A woman's hepatitis C status does not influence obstetric management (SIGN 2006).

Identifying hepatitis C infection during pregnancy can be useful however, for a number of reasons:

- the woman's health status and liver function can be monitored
- she can be given healthy lifestyle advice, including the importance of avoiding alcohol
- she can be given advice to prevent further risk of exposure
- she can be immunised against hepatitis B and hepatitis A
- she can be given information on infection control in the home and elsewhere
- she can be referred for hepatitis C treatment assessment

- the baby can receive appropriate paediatric follow-up, including monitoring for signs and symptoms of hepatitis C in the first year of life, immunisation for hepatitis B and HCV PCR testing.

It is **good practice** therefore to offer the test to pregnant women *at risk of HCV infection* (RCM 2008b).

Risk factors for hepatitis C include:

- History of intravenous drug use, HIV or HBV infection
- Persistent abnormal ALT (liver function test)
- Recipients of blood or blood products, and organ/tissue transplants prior to 1992
- Sexual partner with a history of injecting drug use
- Sexual partner known to have either HIV, HCV or HBV infection
- Unsterile medical or dental procedures abroad where infection control may be poor (i.e. countries other than North America, Australia/New Zealand, and Western Europe)
- Exposure to blood (e.g. through needle stick injury) from someone known to be, or suspected to be, hepatitis C positive
- Unsterile body piercing, tattoos, acupuncture etc

Because testing for hepatitis C during pregnancy is not part of routine screening, the midwife may want to refer the woman to her general practitioner or other HCV testing site or service. If however, the midwife feels competent to do the test, the HCV test can be performed on antenatal booking blood and requested as an additional test on the antenatal screening form. All staff offering the HCV test to pregnant women should follow testing procedure guidelines, which include guidance on pre and post-test discussion topics, and referral for follow-up of mother, and follow-up of baby (if required). Informed consent should be obtained prior to testing.

Mothers found to be **HCV antibody positive and RNA positive** should be offered a referral to a specialist HCV treatment service for follow-up care, whether treatment is considered appropriate or not. Treatment for hepatitis C is now very effective (SIGN 2006). Mothers may choose to start hepatitis C treatment after they have delivered the baby and discontinued breastfeeding.

Babies born to HCV RNA positive mothers, should be referred for paediatric follow-up. The paediatrician will monitor the infant's health, test the infant for signs of infection and, if the infant is found to have acquired the infection (with associated abnormal liver function), refer to gastroenterology for liver disease management. Infants are normally seen by the paediatrician at 3 months and 9 months of age (for HCV RNA testing) and at 18 months of age (for HCV antibody testing). Studies suggest that some infected children (approximately 20–40%) do spontaneously clear the virus (SIGN 2006). The *Children's Liver Disease Foundation* is an organisation that specialises in supporting children with liver disease (www. childliverdisease.org)

Co-infection (HIV and hepatitis)

Co-infection with HIV, HCV and HBV can occur due to shared routes of transmission. The risk of mother-to-child transmission of HCV is twice the rate if co-infected with HIV, even if effective HIV treatment is given (SIGN 2006). C-section is therefore recommended even if there is no indication for a C-section related to HIV (De Ruiter *et al* 2008).

Good practice guidance (Brook *et al* 2010) on blood borne viruses and pregnancy recommends that:
- All HIV positive pregnant women should be screened for hepatitis B and C.
- All HIV positive and HCV infected pregnant women should be vaccinated against HBV if non-immune.
- All HBV and HCV infected pregnant women should be vaccinated against hepatitis A if non-immune.
- All HBV and HCV infected pregnant women should have a discussion on alcohol avoidance and how to reduce the risks of transmission.
- Parenteral and sexual contacts of HCV positive pregnant women should be contacted if possible, in order to offer testing.

Note: Hepatitis B and hepatitis A immunisations can be safely administered during pregnancy or postpartum (Salisbury *et al* 2006 'The Green Book').

Ideally, all women at risk of blood borne viruses should be offered testing before they conceive. Pre-conception advice offered to known HIV positive women who are planning a pregnancy should include a discussion on mother-to-child transmission risks, a full virology screen, screening for STIs, and their medication should be adjusted to a regime that is non-teratogenic. Women who undergo hepatitis C treatment should be advised that the treatment is *contraindicated* during pregnancy and breastfeeding and conception should be avoided for at least four months post-treatment (men six months post-treatment). For further information on family planning care see *Pre-conception care* section.

Maternity care

The next section of the resource book provides information and good practice guidance for maternity care. Maternity care includes:

- pre-conception care
- antenatal care
- intrapartum care
- postnatal care.

This guidance is concise and is intended to complement other relevant publications such as:

- *Antenatal care: routine care for the healthy pregnant women* (NICE 2008)
- *Intrapartum care: care of healthy women and their babies during childbirth* (NICE 2007)
- *Routine postnatal care for women and their babies* (NICE 2006)
- *Care of pregnant women with complex social factors: a model for service provision* (NICE 2010)
- *Antenatal and postnatal mental health: clinical management and service guidance* (NICE 2007)
- *Improving the nutrition of pregnant and breastfeeding mothers and children in low income households* (NICE 2008)
- *Clinical Standards – March 2005: Maternity Services* (NHSQIS 2005)

Pre-conception care

Good health and social circumstances before pregnancy benefits the woman, her unborn baby and the wider family (Scottish Executive 2001). All professionals should routinely ask women whether they have any plans to have a child in the near future, or whether they may be currently pregnant. This questioning needs to be done sensitively as part of the overall assessment and care planning process. Helping a woman prepare and plan for pregnancy and motherhood provides a good opportunity to offer healthy lifestyle and harm reduction education and advice.

All women with drug and alcohol related problems could benefit from receiving information and advice on:

- contraception
- sexual health
- reproductive health
- pre-conception care.

In the UK, the prevalence of drug and alcohol problems is far higher in men than in women (HM Government 2007, Department of Health 2007a). Professionals and agencies in contact with men who use substances should also routinely enquire if they plan to have children, or if their partner is currently pregnant. Family planning, safer sex, the use of condoms, contraception methods, and fertility issues, should be routinely discussed with all men who are sexually active. Men have an important role to play in preventing unplanned and unwanted pregnancies.

Reproductive health and drug use

Reliable information on how drug use affects reproductive health has been difficult to establish and findings are often inconclusive. Theoretically, illicit and dependent drug use can affect fertility in a number of ways, in both women and men (Hepburn 2004a, Wright & Walker 2007).

Substance misuse is associated with poor nutrition and loss of appetite. Significant weight loss can cause amenorrhoea (absent periods) with anovulation (failure to ovulate or produce eggs). Opiates (such as heroin, methadone and DF118) and stimulants (such as amphetamines, cocaine and ecstasy) can interfere with a woman's monthly cycle in this way. Amenorrhoea does not necessarily mean that the woman is unable to conceive (fall pregnant) as she may still be ovulating, so effective contraception to avoid unwanted pregnancies is still required. Irregular or absent periods means that some women may not realise they are pregnant until late in pregnancy when fetal movements are felt, or until other changes are noticed.

Fertility may increase around the time when a woman reduces or comes off drugs or when she starts treatment with substitute drugs, such as methadone. Offering contraceptive advice and pre-conception counselling therefore needs to go hand in hand with the beginning of any drug treatment (Hepburn 2004a).

All professionals can encourage women to attend health care services that provide contraceptive and sexual health advice and care. GPs and family planning clinics will discuss contraceptive options and advise women about how to get emergency contraception if needed. Long-acting reversible contraception (LARC), such as implants, which are effective in reducing unplanned or unwanted pregnancies, should be actively promoted.

Women and men with drug and alcohol problems may plan to conceive or may have an unplanned pregnancy. If pregnancy is planned then pre-conception care can be offered.

Pre-conception advice

Health, social and voluntary sector professionals all have a role to play in providing pre-conception care to women and men with problem substance use. General practitioners are in an ideal position to provide pre-conception care to drug-using women and men who are attending their medical practice for a substitute prescription. If the woman is attending specialist drug or alcohol services then specialist addiction workers have an excellent opportunity to provide pre-conception care. Other workers can address many of the social issues and encourage women and their partners to attend to any health checks that they may need.

Pre-conception care may include a discussion on some or all of the following topics:
- Information on maternity services and the importance of antenatal care
- The woman's past obstetric history, including past pregnancy outcomes and the health and social circumstances of previous children
- The importance of good nutrition and a healthy balanced diet
- The use of Vitamin D supplements and folic acid (to prevent neural tube defects)
- Checking for rubella immunity and vaccination if indicated
- Testing for sexually transmitted diseases if needed e.g. chlamydia
- Testing for blood borne viruses (HIV, hepatitis C and hepatitis B)
- Immunisation for hepatitis B and hepatitis A if required
- Cervical smear if needed
- Screening for toxoplasmosis and cytomegalovirus (if HIV positive or immunosuppressed)
- Review of other conditions e.g. epileptic management and medication, anti-depressant medication
- The importance of good oral hygiene and dental care
- The benefits of breastfeeding
- Healthy lifestyle education, including physical exercise, reducing stress etc

- Options for post-natal contraception and the importance of preventing unwanted pregnancies
- Assessment of other physical and psychological health problems that may affect pregnancy and parenthood i.e. significant illnesses, domestic abuse, past or present mental health problems etc
- Assessment of social circumstances, including such issues as housing, debts and welfare benefits, employment and training, offending behaviour and legal circumstances etc
- Assessment of support networks, including partner, parents, siblings, other family members and friends
- The partner's history of drug/alcohol related problems, including their current use, level of stability if drug dependent, and contact with drug or alcohol treatment services
- Advice on relationships and the transition into parenthood
- Information and advice on child development, parenting skills and child care services.

Pre-conception advice on **drug use** can include:
- The risks associated with smoking during pregnancy and advice on smoking cessation and smoking cessation support services
- The risks of moderate to excessive alcohol use during pregnancy and advice on how to cut down consumption
- Alcohol brief interventions and advice to avoid alcohol for 3 months before conception and during pregnancy
- Information on alcohol services and how to access them
- The risks associated with drug use during pregnancy, in particular illicit drug use and injecting drug use
- The risk of Neonatal Abstinence Syndrome (NAS) in babies born to drug dependent mothers
- The increased risk of SIDS in babies born to mothers who smoke tobacco or take drugs
- Options for drug management during pregnancy and the importance of substitute prescribing and stability for opiate dependent women
- Information on drug services and how to access them
- Information on mother-to-baby transmission of blood borne viruses and how this can be reduced.

All women with a poor obstetric or medical history, or a previous poor fetal or obstetric outcome, or a family history of significant illness should be offered specific pre-conception services (NHSQIS 2005, NICE 2008a). The woman should be encouraged to discuss this with her GP in the first instance.

Further information and advice about sexual health, contraception and family planning can be obtained from the Family Planning Association www.fpa.org.uk

Antenatal care

Receiving good quality antenatal care is known to improve pregnancy and neonatal outcomes, irrespective of continued drug/alcohol use (Broekhuizen *et al* 1992, Department of Health 2007a). All women with problem substance use should be told about the benefits of antenatal care and advised to attend early in pregnancy (NICE 2010a).

Maternity care (for 'low risk' pregnancies) is now primarily community based and midwife managed. Care is 'individualised' and depends on the needs of the individual woman and her circumstances. Midwives follow a 'care pathway' for antenatal and postnatal care, which includes routine antenatal appointments, screening tests and other procedures during pregnancy (depending on parity), parenthood education, preparation for childbirth and postnatal visits. Detailed guidance on routine antenatal care for healthy pregnant women has been published by the National Institute for Health and Clinical Excellence (NICE 2008a) and NHS Quality Improvement Scotland (NHSQIS 2009). Additionally, NICE has published further guidance on the care of pregnant women with complex social factors (NICE 2010a). This includes clinical guidance on the management of pregnant women with drug and alcohol problems and the many special issues which they face.

Community midwives, GPs and consultant obstetricians now jointly manage the care of pregnant women with substance use problems. All women identified as having a drug or alcohol related problem should have a named midwife and a named consultant obstetrician to ensure continuity of care. The consultant obstetrician will see the woman early in pregnancy and will assess and manage any pregnancy complications and/or obstetric risks throughout the pregnancy. Most consultant obstetricians now run outreach clinics in community healthcare centres and can see the woman close to her place of residence. Only a small number of substance-using women need to be managed in 'high risk' clinics in hospital settings by obstetricians, and this is normally for other pregnancy complications (e.g. HIV positive).

All pregnant women receive a copy of *The Pregnancy Book* (Department of Health 2009) or *Ready Steady Baby* book (produced by NHS Health Scotland 2009), which contains comprehensive information on all aspects of pregnancy, childbirth and postnatal care and will help the woman in her decision-making. The GP or midwife will normally give a copy of the book to the woman at first contact after confirmation of pregnancy. At first contact, the healthcare professional will undertake an initial risk assessment and offer early pregnancy care advice.

Hand held maternity records

Record keeping is an integral part of care and assists communication between maternity staff, the woman and others providing care (RCOG *et al* 2008). All professionals involved in a woman's care should ensure that important information is recorded in the woman's maternity record.

All pregnant women now receive a 'woman-held maternity record'. This is normally given to the woman at around 10–12 weeks gestation and she keeps it until she is admitted into hospital for delivery. The woman is encouraged to contribute to her maternity notes if she wishes. Most maternity services now also have complementary electronic recording systems for maternity records. These IT systems are not always accessible to other healthcare staff, for example GPs, so pregnant women with problem substance use should be advised to take their hand held maternity record to other healthcare appointments throughout their pregnancy, so that important information about the woman's pregnancy and her maternity care plan can be seen by other clinicians.

The 'booking appointment'

Pregnant women can either self refer to the midwifery team, or be referred by their GP or other agency. Many areas now have a centralised maternity booking system to assist speedy open access. The booking appointment is normally arranged for 8–12 weeks gestation and is a very important appointment for the woman to attend. At the booking appointment the midwife completes a comprehensive assessment of the woman's needs and will plan pregnancy care with the woman. The midwife also undertakes a risk assessment to take into account any factors that might affect pregnancy outcome and the woman's ability to care for her baby.

At the booking appointment the midwife routinely asks about all drug use, including tobacco, alcohol, illicit drug use, prescribed drugs and the use of over-the-counter medications. Screening and brief interventions for alcohol use are now routinely included in the booking appointment (see section on *Management of substance use during pregnancy*). Any substance use reported by the woman is recorded in the woman's maternity notes. The midwife also asks about mental health problems, domestic abuse and the partner's use of tobacco, alcohol, and drugs.

Women who report drug or alcohol related problems are asked to provide further information so that maternity staff can assess the woman's pattern of substance use, treatment history, social circumstances and likely implications for the pregnancy and neonate. This is normally recorded on an additional information sheet, such as the *Antenatal liaison form (problem substance use)* – see appendix 10, which is included in the woman's notes. This information is then made available to antenatal ward, labour ward, postnatal ward and neonatal unit staff. This enables intrapartum and postnatal care to be co-ordinated and tailored to the special needs of the woman and her baby.

At booking, the community midwife provides information about the risks associated with tobacco, alcohol and drug use during pregnancy and advice about how to minimise any risks. All pregnant women with drug and alcohol related problems should receive user-friendly information such as that contained in the information leaflet *Pregnant... and using drugs and alcohol?* – see appendix 4. Women who are prescribed substitute drugs such as methadone should also be given more detailed information on Neonatal Abstinence Syndrome (NAS) such as that contained in the information leaflet *Caring for a baby with drug withdrawal symptoms* – see appendix 9. The woman and her partner should be given the opportunity to read the information leaflets then discuss any questions or anxieties that they may have in relation to their particular circumstances.

It is important to remember that for some women their drug and alcohol use may come to light for the first time because of their pregnancy care. If this happens there is an excellent opportunity for harm reduction advice and education to be offered and a referral to a drug/alcohol treatment service. This may lead to a change in the woman's substance use. Other women may know they have a drug or alcohol related problem but choose not to disclose this information to health and social care professionals. Some women may acknowledge that they use alcohol or drugs but grossly under-report their use. These women are sometimes identified when problems manifest in the neonate, at which point appropriate treatment and care can be offered.

Many women with drug related problems are already known to drug services and will be on prescribed substitute medication e.g. methadone. Similarly, women with alcohol problems are often known to services and can be offered additional treatment and support throughout the pregnancy. In many areas, especially large urban areas, specialist midwives and/or inter-agency teams have been established to offer enhanced care to women with drug and alcohol problems. In all cases, pregnant women who disclose problem drug or alcohol use should be offered a referral to an appropriate substance misuse service (NICE 2010a).

Routine antenatal screening at booking

At the booking appointment, the community midwife will also offer 'routine antenatal screening'. Blood samples are taken for: HIV, hepatitis B, rubella, syphilis, blood group and a full blood count.

Please note the following regarding hepatitis C:
● Women who are currently injecting drugs or who have a history of injecting drug use may be at risk of hepatitis C. Hepatitis C is also prevalent in populations of people who present with alcohol problems.
● Testing for hepatitis C is not offered routinely, however it should be offered to at risk women (RCM 2008b).

For more detailed information on antenatal testing for HIV, hepatitis B and hepatitis C, and the management of positive women and their babies see '*Blood borne viruses and pregnancy*' section.

Other screening and diagnostic tests

Numerous screening and diagnostic procedures are offered during pregnancy. These are especially important for drug and alcohol using women who may be at increased risk of pregnancy complications. Drug use is associated with an increased risk of intrauterine growth restriction (IUGR) so care should be taken to assess fetal growth by clinical examination, ultrasound and antenatal fetal monitoring. Staff should be careful to explain the reasons for any additional tests sensitively to the woman.

Ultrasound scan is normally arranged for 12 weeks. It is important partly to confirm gestational age, but also to provide the mother (and partner) with a positive experience of the hospital. Substance-using women often worry about fetal abnormality more than any other problem and feel guilty about the damage they may have caused their baby. In general, it is usually possible to be quite reassuring (Johnstone 1998).

Fetal anomaly scanning is now offered to all pregnant women at 20 weeks. If any abnormality is detected the woman is referred to the fetal medicine team for specialist follow-up.

Attendance for fetal monitoring (cardiotocography or CTG) may sometimes be necessary for substance-using women, particularly if growth restriction (IUGR) is established. Please note however, that there may be reduced activity (loss of variability and accelerations) following ingestion of opiates, benzodiazepines and alcohol. Repeat or extended monitoring is sometimes required. The biophysical profile is less affected and will usually be normal even after ingestion of drugs. Another fetal monitoring test, the umbilical artery doppler assessment, can identify vascular problems in the placenta, which can lead to distress or death. This test might be necessary for women who are heavy users of stimulant drugs (such as cocaine or amphetamines) or women in whom IUGR is demonstrated by ultrasound.

Some women drug users (for instance those working in the sex industry) are at higher risk of sexually transmitted and other vaginal infections, which are a risk factor in preterm labour and delivery. It is therefore important to detect and treat all infections during pregnancy. Screening for chlamydia, gonorrhoea, bacterial vaginosis and Group B streptococcus should be considered.

Some women (in particular HIV positive and immuno-compromised women) may also be at greater risk of cervical intraepithelial neoplasia (CIN) and may not have attended for routine cytological screening (cervical smears). Pregnancy can be a good opportunity to attract women into cytological surveillance, certainly in the 1st and early 2nd trimester.

Pregnancy complications

Other complications can occur in substance-using women but not much more frequently than other women, with the exception of women using large amounts of stimulants, such as cocaine, because of the risk of placental abruption (Addis *et al* 2001, Department of Health 2007a).

Preterm labour and delivery is a particular problem that poses a difficult start to mothering and is a significant risk to the baby. It is more common in drug dependent women, particularly those using illicit drugs intravenously or taking short-acting opiates – for example, heroin (Hepburn 2004, Almario *et al* 2009, Department of Health 2007a). Preterm delivery is associated with increased neonatal mortality. Infections also account for some preterm labour episodes so screening is advisable. Pregnant women should be advised to present themselves early if they think they are in preterm labour so that an injection of steroids can be given to help mature the fetal lungs.

Maternal health problems

Good nutrition during pregnancy is important for the development of the baby (NICE 2008a, 2008b, Scottish Government 2011). All pregnant women should be given advice about:
- Eating a healthy balanced diet, including foods rich in iron and calcium.
- Nutritional supplementation (including Vitamin D and folic acid).
- Food hygiene (including how to reduce the risk of food-acquired infections).
- The benefits of breastfeeding.
- The *Healthy Start* Programme.

A good source of information about nutrition and diet during pregnancy can be obtained from the *Food Standards Agency* (FSA) which can be accessed online. NICE (2008b) have also produced guidance on improving the nutrition of pregnant and breastfeeding women and children in low-income households.

Pregnant women are routinely tested for anaemia at their antenatal appointments and will be prescribed iron if necessary. They should be advised to take a folic acid supplement (400 micrograms) for the first 12 weeks of pregnancy to prevent neural tube defects as well as a daily supplement of Vitamin D (10 micrograms) during pregnancy and whilst breastfeeding (Scottish Government 2011).

Constipation is very common in pregnancy and can be exacerbated by opiate use, so women should be advised to increase their fibre intake and drink more water. Nausea and vomiting in pregnancy is common but does not have harmful effects on pregnancy outcome (NICE 2008a). However, it can severely impact on quality of life, and some drug users may report difficulty in keeping down their methadone, especially in the first 16–20 weeks of pregnancy. If this is the case, advise the woman to consult with their prescriber to consider ways of reducing these effects. Ginger, wrist acupressure, and splitting the daily dose of methadone can sometimes help. Sipping methadone slowly over a period of an hour or so may also help.

Poor general health and drug use can lead to respiratory problems, including chest infections and asthma. Repeated injections over years destroys peripheral veins, often leaving 'track marks' so venous access may be limited even in women who stopped injecting drugs years before (Hepburn 2004a).

Good dental care in pregnancy is especially important. All pregnant women with problem substance use should be encouraged to attend their dentist for a check up so that they can get any necessary dental treatment and avoid dental decay and infections in pregnancy (Hepburn 2004b). Severe dental problems are commonly associated with opiate use. This is made worse by the high sugar content and acidity of methadone (Department of Health 2007a). Sugar free methadone is available on prescription, but the acid content is similar to the normal preparation. Advise all women to brush their teeth with fluoride toothpaste *before* they take their methadone and rinse their mouth afterwards with water. Sugar free chewing gum will also help clear the methadone from their mouths. Women tend to suffer increased gum problems during pregnancy, which can show itself as bleeding gums. This can be more serious in women with substance use problems and progress to acute and very painful infections.

Maternity benefits and allowances

All pregnant women should be given information on benefits and allowances that are available during and after pregnancy. These include:

- Entitlement to free NHS prescriptions and free NHS dental treatment throughout pregnancy and for one year after the birth of their baby
- The 'Sure Start Maternity Grant' is available to women on a low income who are (or whose partners are) claiming certain benefits or tax credits. It is worth up to £500 and is tax free. A midwife, health visitor or doctor can sign the application form (which confirms the woman has received health education and antenatal care).
- Entitlement to 'Healthy Start' vouchers (if on a low income) which can be used to buy free milk, fruit, vegetables, infant formula and vitamins.

Further information on benefits is available from:
● Directgov www.direct.gov.uk
● Healthy Start www.healthystart.nhs.uk
● Social Security booklet *A guide to maternity benefits* (Department for Work and Pensions 2010).

Preparation for parenthood

All pregnant women and their partners are offered antenatal classes for 'parent education' and this normally starts at around 28–32 weeks gestation. Group and individual sessions can be organised and are jointly run by midwives and health visitors. All parent education sessions are community-based. They normally include information regarding pregnancy, childbirth, infant feeding, parenting and child development. However, they do encompass broader supportive measures that help women and their partners to understand and explore their own social, emotional, psychological and physical needs during this time (NICE 2008a). The aim of parent education is to provide an opportunity for parents to develop self-awareness and confidence in their abilities, to have a positive experience of the birth, and to adjust more successfully to parenthood and the changes that parenthood brings.

Parent education is especially important for women and men with problem substance use and for first time mothers and fathers. For further information contact your local community midwifery team. Professionals should encourage parents to attend these sessions as many people with problem substance use have not had positive parenting role models and attendance is often poor.

Risk assessment during pregnancy

All professionals working with pregnant women with substance use problems should have a clear understanding of the concept of risk assessment to ensure safety for mother and baby. Risk should be continuously assessed throughout the pregnancy, taking into account that risk status is dynamic and may change over time (NICE 2008a).

Significant risk factors that would indicate the need for further assessment and intervention might include:
● Poor obstetric and pregnancy outcome history
● Poor maternal health/significant illness/HIV, hepatitis C or hepatitis B
● High alcohol consumption (including binge drinking) or alcohol dependence

- Injecting drug use or illicit (non-prescribed) drug use
- Neonate at risk of developing Neonatal Abstinence Syndrome (NAS), or previous baby with NAS
- History of severe mental health problem (e.g. schizophrenia, bipolar disorder, postnatal depression/puerperal psychosis, eating disorder)
- Learning difficulties/cognitive impairment which is likely to affect parenting capacity
- Domestic abuse/parental conflict
- Criminal justice involvement/member of family a sex offender
- Teenage pregnancy/unsupported pregnancy
- Homelessness and insecure/unsuitable/unsafe accommodation
- Ethnic minority, refugee or asylum seeker
- Other significant social concerns (e.g. lack of necessary household material possessions, significant debts or financial difficulties, sex industry worker)
- Existing children on 'at risk' register/accommodated by local authority
- Recorded history of previous parenting or child care concerns.

Remember that many of the above risk factors may be applicable to the **father/ woman's partner** rather than the woman herself, and should be responded to in the same way.

Not registered with a GP

Pregnant women who are not registered with a general practitioner should be encouraged to do so as soon as possible. If the woman experiences any difficulty registering with a GP then she should be advised to contact the local Primary Care Trust or Health Care Partnership to request a GP be 'allocated' to her. Requests should be made in writing. Advise the woman to complete the proforma letter (see appendix 11) and send to the local Primary Care Services Department.

Homelessness or housing problems

It is important that the woman finds suitable accommodation in time for her to prepare for the birth of her baby. Homelessness creates additional stress for the woman and can make attendance for antenatal care difficult. Good liaison and care planning are required to ensure agencies are working together. Pregnant women also need to engage early with the health visiting service who will encourage the family to move towards accessing mainstream services once they are in stable accommodation.

Pregnant women who are homeless or in temporary accommodation, can register with a GP in a 'homeless practice'. These GP practices, available in urban areas, normally have additional health and social care staff who work together to assist vulnerable adults and children. Midwives who work with patients registered in homeless GP practices will arrange to visit the woman at the clinic or in temporary accommodation.

Domestic abuse

Domestic abuse (also known as gender-based violence) is closely associated with substance use, particularly alcohol use (Cleaver *et al* 2010, Barnish 2004, BMA 2007b). It can have a harmful, sometimes even life-threatening, impact on the physical and mental wellbeing of both mother and baby and is a serious criminal, social and medical problem (Department of Health 2005, BMA 2007b, RCM 2009). Domestic abuse can include a wide range of physical (e.g. hitting, kicking, restraining), sexual (including rape and coercion), psychological (verbal bullying, undermining, social isolation) and financial (e.g. withholding money) abuses. Domestic abuse can also be perpetrated via emails, text and telephone messages.

Conclusive evidence has demonstrated that pregnancy, far from being a time of peace and safety, may trigger or exacerbate male violence in the home (RCM 2009). Domestic abuse is widespread and under reported and the level of repeat incidence is high. It is estimated that a third of domestic abuse starts or escalates during pregnancy (Department of Health 2005). Violence may also increase following the birth of a child or when a woman tries to end a relationship (Barnish 2004). Domestic abuse during pregnancy is associated with increased rates of miscarriage, low birth weight, premature birth, fetal injury and fetal death (BMA 2007b). Domestic abuse can have an indirect effect on the fetus and developing baby, because it is associated with increased maternal smoking, alcohol consumption, and stress, and women being prevented from seeking or receiving proper antenatal or postnatal care by their abusive partners (BMA 2007b).

All midwives routinely enquire about domestic abuse as part of their antenatal and postnatal risk assessment. To encourage disclosure, all pregnant women should have at least one consultation with a healthcare professional during the pregnancy which is not attended by the partner or any other family member (BMA 2007b).

Where abuse is suspected, midwives should further ask the woman about abuse explicitly but carefully and sensitively (RCM 2009). Women who disclose domestic abuse should be given advice and support on how and where to get help. Details of services that offer psychological support as well as refuge should be offered. Relevant addresses and telephone numbers should be made easily accessible to enable women to get help with or without the support and knowledge of health and social care staff. Where disclosure is made, referral to appropriate services and any other action deemed necessary should be undertaken.

It is important to note that domestic abuse is considered a child protection issue because the welfare of the unborn child, newborn infant and other children living in the home could be at risk (HM Government 2010, Cleaver *et al* 2010).

Health care staff should refer to the following guidance for further information on how to respond to domestic abuse:

- Department of Health (2009) *Improving safety, Reducing harm: Children, young people and domestic violence: A practical toolkit for front-line practitioners.* London, Department of Health.
- Department of Health (2005) *Responding to domestic abuse: a handbook for healthcare professionals.*
- Scottish Executive (2003) *Responding to domestic abuse: guidelines for health care workers in NHS Scotland.*
- HM Government (2010) *Working together to safeguard children: a guide to inter-agency working to safeguard and promote the welfare of children.*

Parental mental health problems

Mental health problems and alcohol and drug problems are closely associated. Up to 60% of heavy drinkers and dependent drug users reporting moderate to severe incapacity as a result of co-morbid conditions such as anxiety, depression, post traumatic stress disorder, bipolar disorder and psychotic illnesses e.g. schizophrenia (Department of Health 2007a). It is important to identify pregnant women and fathers-to-be who have mental health issues early in pregnancy and ensure they receive appropriate treatment and care for their 'dual diagnosis'. For information on the obstetric management of women with mental health problems and the neonatal management of infants exposed to antipsychotic medication during pregnancy and breastfeeding see *Antenatal and postnatal mental health: clinical management and service guidance* (NICE 2007a).

Both parental mental health problems and parental substance use are associated with an increased risk of poor parenting capacity and child maltreatment (Tunnard 2002a,2002b, 2004). Analysis of serious case reviews have found parental mental health to be a factor in a high proportion of cases (approximately 30% of fatal child abuse cases), and more so when parental substance use is also a presenting factor (Brandon *et al* 2008, 2009). Combined adversities e.g. depression, alcohol and drug problems, violence, homelessness, and an infant with special needs, will provide a complex array of stressors that will require careful multi-disciplinary and multi-agency management. Involvement of the perinatal mental health service may be required. For further guidance on the management of children and families affected by parental mental health problems see *Think child, think parent, think family: a guide to parental mental health and child welfare* (SCIE 2009).

Neonate at risk of Neonatal Abstinence Syndrome (NAS)

It is important to discuss the possibility of Neonatal Abstinence Syndrome (NAS) with all drug dependent women and their partners at an early stage. They need to know that NAS is usually easily managed but that the baby will need some special care as well as their support, understanding and patience. Having a baby who develops severe withdrawal symptoms can be very distressing for parents, but if properly looked after the baby will make a full recovery (Johnstone 1998, American Academy of Paediatrics 1998). It is important to document in the woman's maternity notes that the baby is at risk of developing NAS. This notification or 'alert' in the woman's notes should ensure that the baby is not discharged home without appropriate postnatal care.

The service user information leaflet *Caring for a baby with drug withdrawal symptoms* (see appendix 9), provides detailed information for parents. This leaflet should be given to all drug dependent women and their partners at the booking appointment. They should be given an opportunity to read the leaflet and to discuss their birth plan and care of their baby with the midwife/obstetrician and health visitor. For more detailed information see section '*Neonatal Abstinence Syndrome (NAS)*'.

Child welfare concerns

A risk assessment may identify concerns about the ability of the woman (or her partner) to look after their infant. If this is the case, then it is important to address these concerns with the woman and her partner at an early stage. All professionals in contact with pregnant women have a responsibility to act if they believe that the baby will be at risk of harm. A pro-active and early intervention approach is more likely to result in a positive outcome for mother, baby and family.

Professionals should make themselves familiar with:
- Local inter-agency child protection procedures and risk assessment frameworks.
- HM Government (2010) *Working together to safeguard children: a guide to inter-agency working to safeguard and promote the welfare of children.*
- NICE (2009) *When to suspect child maltreatment: Clinical Guideline*
- Scottish Government (2010) *National guidance on child protection in Scotland*
- Scottish Executive (2003) *Getting Our Priorities Right: Good Practice Guidance for Working with Children and Families affected by Substance Misuse*

These documents contain important information for professionals, including:
- The guiding principles of safeguarding children
- The legal framework for child protection
- Professional roles and responsibilities in relation to protecting the welfare of children
- Guidance on information sharing and confidentiality
- The signs and symptoms of physical abuse, neglect, non organic failure to thrive, emotional abuse and sexual abuse
- The impact of parental problem substance use on infants and children
- The referral process for dealing with child care concerns and child protection issues
- A checklist of information to be collated concerning problem substance use and its impact on parenting
- The practicalities of protecting and supporting the children of problem substance users
- A helpful contact list of professionals who have expertise in child protection.

For more detailed guidance on dealing with child care concerns see section *'Assessing parenting capacity and child care risk during pregnancy'.*

Intrapartum care (labour and childbirth)

The vast majority of labours and deliveries will be straightforward in drug and alcohol using women and thus their care will be similar to most other woman (Hepburn 2004a, Wright & Walker 2007). There are however, a few important factors to consider. These should be read in conjunction with other clinical guidelines on intrapartum care which have been published – for example, NICE (2007b) *Intrapartum care for healthy women and their babies*.

Currently, most intrapartum care is provided by midwives who staff the labour suite on rotation. The pregnant woman may see a number of different midwives if she has several antenatal episodes in the labour suite (for instance for preterm labour) and her named midwife in the community may not be the one who delivers her baby.

The obstetrician and paediatrician are kept informed during labour, but they are not the key professionals unless there are complications (for instance, preterm delivery).

Midwives delivering intrapartum care should make sure they read the woman's hand held maternity records and any other confidential or 'sensitive' information held in admissions. The *antenatal liaison form (problem substance use)* provides detailed information on the woman's drug/alcohol use, medication, pharmacist and key professionals and services involved in her care (see appendix 10). This is a helpful tool to record essential information for busy labour ward staff to read and consider in terms of the woman's management during childbirth.

Maternity hospital policy

The woman, her partner and family all need to understand the hospital priority for a safe pregnancy and childbirth experience. This means zero tolerance of illicit drug use on hospital premises, clear limits on the conduct of herself and any visitors, and zero tolerance for abusive, threatening or aggressive behaviour. If necessary, visitors will be removed from the building and barred from returning.

Substitute prescribed drugs are dispensed by the hospital pharmacy but only after the dose of medication has been checked with the prescribing doctor and any community prescriptions have been cancelled with the pharmacist. This means that hospital staff will need to know the name, address and telephone number of the prescribing doctor and pharmacy. This information should be written clearly in the notes. The woman should remember to take any supply of medication into hospital with her, as it will not be replaced if it has already been dispensed in the community. On discharge, the hospital will notify the prescribing doctor when the next dose of medication is due to be dispensed from the community.

Pain relief during childbirth

Women who use drugs may be fearful of labour and childbirth and worry that they will not get adequate pain relief (Hepburn 2004a). It is very important that adequate pain relief is given and the midwife establishes a good rapport with the woman, offering reassurance and support when required. It is a good idea to discuss pain relief options in the antenatal period so that the woman feels confident that she will be well cared for and treated like any other woman in labour.

Prescribed medication should be dispensed as normal during labour. Substitution treatment with methadone does not provide pain relief (Hepburn 2004a). Opioid receptors may be saturated so higher doses or more frequent injections of diamorphine may be needed. There is usually a low threshold for an epidural anaesthesia and many drug dependent women opt for this pain management approach.

Caesarean section is no more likely than in the normal population and having a history of problem drug use should not be considered a contraindication to having a PCA pump (patient controlled analgesia pump) following caesarean section (Siney 1999). Post delivery pain relief should be the same as for every other woman, although higher doses may be required.

Complications of childbirth

In women with a history of injecting drug use, venous access may be poor and antenatal referral to an anaesthetist may be required. Where labour is straightforward, no intravenous line is required. However, if it appears that there might be complications, it is sometimes better to establish an intravenous line electively shortly after admission, rather than be faced with the task in an emergency situation (Johnstone 1998).

There may be placental insufficiency in pregnancies of drug-using women, leading to an increased risk of intrapartum hypoxia, fetal distress and meconium staining (Department of Health 2007a). Meconium aspiration is common and is associated with fetal distress secondary to periods of intra-uterine drug withdrawal. Some babies will be growth restricted so there should be careful surveillance during labour. Maternity staff should follow hospital guidelines for obstetric and neonate management for meconium staining.

High dose benzodiazepine use in the mother can result in the newborn showing signs of intoxication at birth that include: poor sucking, poor reflexes, hypotonia (low muscle tone), hypothermia (low body temperature), a feeble cry and low APGAR scores. Severely affected neonates may require vigorous resuscitation at birth because of respiratory depression. Women who are anxious about childbirth should be warned not to 'self medicate' with non-prescribed benzodiazepines (e.g. Valium®) before they admit themselves for delivery.

Please note: Labour ward staff must not use naloxone (an opiate antagonist) to reverse opioid induced respiratory depression in neonates as this will induce an abrupt opiate withdrawal crisis. Use supportive measures or ventilation if necessary.

Postpartum care in hospital

After delivery, the labour ward midwife should liaise with staff in the postnatal ward to ensure continuity of care. The named midwife in the community should also be informed of the delivery. This is particularly important if the woman has delivered preterm. Maternity staff providing intrapartum care should complete details of the birth and outcome of pregnancy – for example, by using the *Postnatal liaison form (problem substance use)* – see appendix 10.

Drug dependent women are normally asked to stay in hospital for three days (72 hours) following the birth of their baby. This is because the baby needs to be observed for signs and symptoms of Neonatal Abstinence Syndrome (NAS), which normally develop within this time period – see section on *Neonatal Abstinence Syndrome* for further information.

Confinement in hospital can be a threatening or difficult experience for some substance-using women. Staff should take care to ensure respect and privacy by being discreet about the administration of any medications (e.g. methadone) so that the woman's drug use is not exposed to other patients or visiting relatives who might not know about her drug use.

Soon after delivery, mother and baby should be transferred to the postnatal ward where they can 'room in' together and have 'skin-to-skin' contact. Separating mother and baby should be avoided if at all possible (Department of Health 2007a). 'Skin-to-skin' contact will help the baby relax and sleep, regulate their body temperature, steady their breathing, help with mother-infant bonding and will help get breastfeeding off to a good start (NICE 2008a).

Women who have a history of alcohol related problems (who remain in the postnatal ward) can be observed for maternal symptoms of alcohol withdrawal (which typically occur around 48 hours post delivery), in which case appropriate medication may be required (Wright & Walker 2007).

Ideally, discussion about the need for postnatal contraception should have been instigated in the antenatal period rather than at the discharge planning meeting. Many women with problem substance use may not be able to address their reproductive and sexual health needs adequately. Planning contraception for the postnatal period involves considering 'what, how and when?' to start using contraception – for example, combined oral contraceptive pill, progestogen-only pill, 'Depo-Provera®', 'Implanon®', the coil or long acting reversible contraception (LARC). Advice on choices also varies depending on whether the woman is breastfeeding or not. Condoms are normally recommended for the first 48 hours post-delivery or for the first few weeks following delivery until hormonal contraception has been started.

After 72 hours on the postnatal ward, mother and baby can be safely discharged home, provided the baby is well enough and the care-giving environment has been assessed as being safe and nurturing. On discharge, all women are given a 'discharge pack' which contains helpful information leaflets on caring for their baby.

In circumstances where the mother insists on taking an early discharge, she should be seen by the paediatrician and asked to sign a form that states she is taking the baby home against medical advice. If there is any uncertainty about the mother or father's parenting capacity then social work should be informed and an urgent assessment of the situation should result in a decision about the discharge of the infant. In rare cases, the mother may take her own discharge and leave the baby in hospital. If this happens, the baby will be transferred to the Neonatal Unit (NNU)/ Special Care Baby Unit (SCBU) for continued monitoring.

Infant feeding

Increasing breastfeeding rates, especially in areas of deprivation, is a key public health priority and is embedded in Infant Feeding Strategies. Breastfeeding can make a major contribution to an infant's long-term health and development, reducing the incidence of conditions such as gastroenteritis, eczema and asthma. It is also linked to better health outcomes for the mother, including cutting down the risks of breast and ovarian cancer, osteoporosis and obesity (WHO 2003, Department of Health 2003).

Much confusion surrounds the issue of whether a woman should breastfeed her baby when continuing to take drugs. Parents should be informed that the benefits of breastfeeding normally outweigh the disadvantages, even with continued substance use (Department of Health 2007a).

Breast milk is the best form of nutrition for infants (Department of Health 2003). The World Health Organisation (2003) recommends that infants should be exclusively breastfed for the first 6 months of life in order to achieve optimal growth, development and health. Thereafter, infants should receive nutritionally adequate and safe complementary foods in addition to breastfeeding for up to 2 years or beyond.

All drug-using mothers should be encouraged to breastfeed unless there are definitive medical or social reasons not to breastfeed. Decisions on safety should be made on a case-by-case basis, after weighing up the benefits and risks of breastfeeding, by referring to the evidence (published research), and by taking into account pharmacological principles, harm reduction strategies and child welfare concerns. Where possible, breastfeeding should always be promoted and the woman's wishes respected.

Please note: It is essential that those involved in discussing the benefits and risks of breastfeeding with substance-using women are sufficiently trained and competent to do so. Inaccurate, incomplete or inconsistent advice is likely to undermine the woman's confidence, confuse her decision-making, and may cause unnecessary concern and upset.

Breastfeeding is NOT recommended if the mother is:
● HIV positive − because of the risk of mother-to-child HIV transmission.

Women should be advised that there may be risks involved in breastfeeding if she is:
● Injecting drugs − because of the risk of blood borne virus transmission.
● Using psychostimulant drugs such as cocaine, crack cocaine, amphetamines, methamphetamine or ecstasy − because of risk of impaired functioning in the mother and the potential effects on the infant including insomnia, irritability and feeding problems.

- Using illicit (street) drugs on a regular basis such as heroin and/or benzodiazepines (e.g. diazepam) – because of the risk of impaired functioning in the mother and sedation effects on the infant.
- Drinking alcohol in addition to taking other central nervous system (CNS) depressant drugs such as opiates and benzodiazepines – because of the risk of impaired functioning in the mother and sedation effects on the infant.

Breastfeeding advice and care

Although breastfeeding is generally recommended, all pregnant women with drug and/or alcohol problems should discuss the benefits and risks of breastfeeding with their healthcare provider – usually the midwife, obstetrician or GP providing antenatal care. At the booking appointment (normally around 8–12 weeks gestation), a discussion on breastfeeding should be initiated (NICE 2008a).

It is important to note that the majority of substance-using women are polydrug users. That is, they usually take a combination of different drugs all at the same time or over time. Many will report that they smoke tobacco and cannabis, drink alcohol, take methadone or other opiates (e.g. heroin or dihydrocodeine), benzodiazepines (e.g. diazepam) and stimulant drugs (e.g. cocaine or amphetamines). It is important to establish what drugs the woman is taking, or is likely to take, her pattern of drug use, how she is taking the drugs (e.g. orally or by injection), and her drug treatment plan – in order to determine the risks that her drug use may pose for breastfeeding and to inform the discussion, which should always seek to promote breastfeeding and minimise the risks.

In addition to moving opiate-dependent women onto prescribed medications, for example methadone, and offering additional support, specialist assessment and care by a drug/alcohol service throughout the antenatal period is advised – see *'Management of substance use during pregnancy'* section, and Department of Health (2007a) clinical guidelines. Further support for substance-misusing parents is also available through the antenatal multidisciplinary and interagency meetings which are normally held around 28 weeks gestation.

By 32 weeks gestation or earlier if possible, breastfeeding information, including good management practices, should be given, as outlined in the UNICEF UK 'Baby Friendly Initiative'. If the woman has decided to breastfeed, she should be given advice about the importance of:

- Vitamin D and folic acid intake whilst pregnant and breastfeeding

- Eating well (see *The Pregnancy Book,* Department of Health 2009)
- Skin-to-skin contact after delivery.
- Positioning and attachment of baby on breast.
- Baby-led feeding and feeding cues.
- Rooming-in.
- Avoidance of formula supplements (unless clinically indicated).
- Avoidance of the use of teats.
- Timing of breast feeds in relation to substance intake.
- Advice about weaning and the importance of maintaining breast milk supply if mixed feeding (formula and breastfeeding) is commenced.
- Follow-up advice and support from the midwife, health visitor and GP.
- Clear advice NOT TO SHARE A BED with the baby should be given to all parents who smoke tobacco, drink alcohol or take psychoactive drugs (prescribed or illicit).

Benefits of breastfeeding
- Good for mother and baby from a psychological point of view (promotes bonding and care-giving, mother-infant interactions and secure attachment).
- Good for baby from an immunological point of view (helps prevent infections in infancy and promotes the long term health of the child).
- Good for mother in terms of her long term health.
- Breastfeeding may reduce risk of Sudden Infant Death Syndrome (SIDS).
- Breastfeeding may reduce severity of baby withdrawal symptoms – Neonatal Abstinence Syndrome (NAS).

Patient information/booklets include:
- *'Off to a good start: all you need to know about breastfeeding your baby'*, NHS Health Scotland (2009)
- All pregnant women are offered a free DVD *'From bump to breastfeeding',* a copy of *'The Pregnancy Book'* or *'Ready Steady Baby'* and can access information on www.breastfeeding.nhs.uk

Please note: Individually tailored help for women with limited access to written materials (because of language, capacity or impairment issues) may be required.

Further information for professionals includes: Hoddinott *et al* (2008), and *Good practice and innovation in breastfeeding* (Department of Health 2004).

Potential risks

Decisions about breastfeeding (or continuing to breastfeed) when smoking, drinking alcohol, taking medications or illicit drugs, involve more than a consideration of whether or not the substance/s appear in the mother's milk.

Very few drugs are contraindicated for breastfeeding mothers (Lee 2007). Nearly all drugs pass into human milk, but only in very small amounts – usually < 1% of the maternal dose (Hale 2008). Whilst some drugs do cause problems for infants (even in tiny doses), this is not the case for the vast majority of drugs. Health professionals should seek advice from their local Drug (Medicine) Information Service/pharmacist if they have any queries. Ideally such queries should be made during pregnancy to allow for planning.

Concerns regarding the effects of drugs in lactation may arise because of the potential effects on the mother, potential short and long-term effects on the infant and/or potential effects on milk supply (Lee 2007, Hale 2008).

- Potential effects on the mother depend on her stability of drug use (if she is on methadone for example), the types of substances she is taking, her mental state and behaviour, her ability to manage and sustain a breastfeeding schedule, and the stability of her personal and social circumstances as a whole.
- Potential effects on the infant depend on the type of drug and amount of drug in the milk, its bioavailability and drug side effect profile, the volume of milk consumed and the infant's ability to clear the drug.
- The infant's health and wellbeing should be considered – for example, preterm, very low birth weight and/or sick infants may require a heightened level of monitoring due to the potential for slower clearance of the drug.
- Some drugs may increase or decrease milk production (supply) and affect milk fat concentrations, hence the nutritional intake of the infant.

Methadone and other opiate substitutes

Methadone is NOT a contraindication to breastfeeding (Department of Health 2007a, Hale 2008). Prescribed methadone is safer than non-prescribed drug use, intermittent drug use or rapid withdrawal. Professionals should encourage opiate-dependent women who are prescribed methadone to breastfeed, taking into consideration the issues addressed in this guidance.

Methadone-maintained mothers who choose to breastfeed should aim to keep their drug use as stable as possible, their prescribed dose as low as possible (whilst maintaining stability) and should monitor their infant for signs of over-sedation and breathing difficulties (Department of Health 2007a). Successful establishment of breastfeeding is in itself a marker of adequate stability of drug use (Scottish Executive 2003).

It is important to reassure mothers (and their partners) that the actual amount of methadone passed to the baby through breast milk is minimal and unlikely to have any adverse (neurobehavioural) effects on the infant (Jansson *et al* 2008a, Jansson *et al* 2008b, McCarthy & Posey 2000). Studies on nursing mothers who are enrolled in methadone maintenance programmes have found low milk:plasma ratios, and have assessed relative infant doses as < 0.2 mg/day on average, regardless of the mother's methadone dose (Begg *et al* 2001, Blinick *et al* 1975, Geraghty *et al* 1997, Jansson *et al* 2004, Jansson *et al* 2008a, McCarthy & Posey 2000, Pocock 2008, Wojnar-Horton *et al* 1997).

Evidence suggests that peak concentrations of methadone in breast milk vary, and occur between 1 to 6 hours after the mother takes her daily dose (Begg *et al* 2001, Blinick *et al* 1975, Jansson *et al* 2004, McCarthy & Posey 2000). Mothers may want to time their breastfeeding in order to avoid peak concentration times, however this is often impractical (especially when feeding on demand every 2–4 hours) and it is also NOT necessary, as feeding during times of peak concentration will have little effect on the breastfed infant (Jansson *et al* 2008a).

The small amount of drug passed to the infant through breast milk may ameliorate drug withdrawal symptoms (NAS) in newborn infants (Department of Health 2007a). Delayed onset of symptoms, less severe symptoms, reduced requirement for pharmacological treatment and reduced length of infant hospital stay have been reported (Abdel-Latif *et al* 2006, Malpas *et al* 1997).

Even so, parents should be advised that breastfeeding will not necessarily prevent the infant developing drug withdrawal symptoms (NAS). All parents whose babies are at risk of developing NAS should be adequately prepared – see section '*Neonatal Abstinence Syndrome*'. Breastfeeding mothers on methadone (or benzodiazepines) whose infants develop NAS may need extra breastfeeding support because infants with NAS can have feeding difficulties and specific nutritional needs (e.g. increased calorie intake).

Other drugs, such as dihydrocodeine (DF118), buprenorphine (Subutex®) and buprenorphine/naloxone (Suboxone®) are sometimes prescribed for opioid dependence. Opiate-dependent pregnant women are normally NOT commenced on these substitute treatments, as methadone is the preferred option. However, for those who have been stabilised on these medications during pregnancy and wish to breastfeed, an individual risk-benefit analysis to inform decision-making should be undertaken by the prescriber. Due to the lack of evidence of the effects of these drugs on breastfed infants, manufacturers' advice is to avoid, although expert consensus opinion on *Subutex®* and *Suboxonef* states that any effects of these medications on the breastfed infant is likely to be minimal and that breastfeeding is NOT contraindicated (Center for Substance Abuse Treatment 2004, Hale 2008). There is some evidence to suggest that buprenorphine is poorly absorbed by infants via the oral route, is safe and effective in pregnancy and may help to reduce the incidence and severity of NAS (Center for Substance Abuse Treatment 2004, Johnson *et al* 2003a, Jones *et al* 2010, Fischer *et al* 2006). There is insufficient evidence on the use of high dose dihydrocodeine during lactation to provide more definitive guidance.

The key issue for women who want to remain on these substitute medications whilst breastfeeding is that they understand that the safety of these drugs, especially in the amounts that they may be taking, have not yet been fully evaluated.

Prescribed benzodiazepines

Some drug dependent women are also prescribed benzodiazepines (usually diazepam at dosages of 30 mgs per day or less). Diazepam and other benzodiazepines are excreted into breast milk, albeit at relatively low levels (McElhatton 1994). Manufacturers' advice on the use of diazepam whilst breastfeeding is to avoid if possible. There is a lack of research on benzodiazepine-dependent mothers who breastfeed, but if such women wish to breastfeed, and their benzodiazepine use is stable, they may be supported to do so, so long as a risk-benefit analysis has been undertaken and the potential benefits outweigh the risks. Potential risks include lethargy, sedation and poor suckling (Hale 2008). Advise mothers to keep their dose of diazepam as low as possible whilst breastfeeding and to monitor the infant for signs of over-sedation and low milk intake/poor weight gain.

Alcohol

Alcohol is freely excreted into breast milk (Lee 2007). It can reduce milk production (supply), it can change the taste and smell of milk, alter the infant's sleep pattern, affect the infant's digestion and potentially reduce infant intake (Mennella & Beauchamp 1991, Mennella & Gerrish 1998, NHS Health Scotland 2009).

If a woman chooses to drink alcohol during lactation, then she should be advised to consume no more than one or two units, once or twice a week (NHS Health Scotland 2009). Binge drinking, chronic alcohol use or combining alcohol with other drug use whilst breastfeeding is NOT recommended.

Alcohol levels in breast milk peak around 30–60 minutes after a drink. Alcohol passes freely from the milk into the plasma compartment over time, so a single drink (1 unit) would clear completely from the milk after 2–3 hours (provided the woman does not continue to drink). Mothers can express milk before drinking alcohol or they can avoid breastfeeding for a couple of hours after consuming alcohol (1 or 2 units), to ensure alcohol levels in the milk have diminished.

Tobacco

Breastfeeding should be encouraged regardless of whether the woman is a smoker or not. Although the standard advice given to breastfeeding women is to avoid smoking where possible, smoking is NOT a contraindication to breastfeeding. Research suggests that breastfeeding is still the healthier option for both mother and baby than formula (bottle) feeding (Lee 2007, Hale 2008).

Mothers who choose to smoke should be aware that tobacco smoking may decrease milk production (supply) and lower milk fat concentration (Hale 2008). Nicotine is present in breast milk and can cause gastric irritation for the infant (Shenassa & Brown 2004). Where possible, mothers should allow at least 20 minutes to elapse after smoking a cigarette before they breastfeed, so the amount of nicotine in the breast milk is reduced. Advise mothers, fathers or any others against smoking in the home, particularly in the same room as the infant. Smoking cessation advice, nicotine patches or chewing gum should be offered along with support to attend smoking cessation sessions or 1:1 support – see 'Management of substance use during pregnancy' section.

Cannabis

Despite its widespread use, the effects of cannabis (marijuana) on infants who are breastfed are poorly understood. Cannabis is excreted into breast milk and its metabolite, Tetrahydrocannabinol (THC) can accumulate due to its high fat solubility. With regular or heavy maternal use, the breastfed infant may become unsettled and demand frequent feeding. One study (Ashley & Little 1990) found infants exposed to marijuana through breast milk showed a delay in motor development at 1 year. Where possible, cannabis use should be avoided whilst breastfeeding. However, mothers who use cannabis should not be discouraged from breastfeeding.

Concerns about additional substance use whilst breastfeeding

If a breastfeeding woman takes illicit drugs (or an excessive amount of alcohol) and is worried about the possible effects on the infant she can express and discard her breast milk, seek advice from a health professional, and resume breastfeeding after the substance has cleared (approximately 12–48 hours later, depending on the substance taken and her circumstances). Because of the well-documented benefits of human milk to child health, the risk of interruption or cessation of breastfeeding must be carefully weighed up against the necessity and the risks posed by the drug use under question. Relapse prevention support should be an integral part of the woman's care plan.

If a breastfeeding mother is starting a prescription for methadone (or other substitute medication) for the first-time or is increasing the dose, she should be advised to monitor the infant closely for signs of behaviour change, sedation and breathing difficulties. Breastfeeding mothers who notice that their infant is sedated or has breathing problems should seek medical advice immediately. Every effort should be made to ensure the mother is on a stable dose of methadone (and/or other substitute medication) well before the baby is born.

Sudden Infant Death Syndrome (SIDS)

Babies exposed to tobacco, drugs and alcohol during pregnancy (and after they are born) are at increased risk of SIDS (Kandall *et al* 1993, Friend *et al* 2004, American Academy of Pediatrics 2005). Strategies to reduce the risk of SIDS need to be discussed with all substance-using mothers and fathers – see *Reducing the risk of cot death* (Department of Health 2009d).

Bed-sharing, combined with smoking, alcohol and/or other drug use is associated with an increased risk of SIDS (Blair *et al* 1999, American Academy of Paediatrics 2005, McKenna & McDade 2005, Horsley *et al* 2007). Along with a discussion on the benefits and risks of breastfeeding, and breastfeeding methods, substance-using parents should be advised NOT to bed-share with their infant and to always place their infant to sleep on their back (American Academy of Paediatrics 2005).

Mothers who are under the influence of drugs or alcohol are likely to be less responsive to the needs of their infant because of impaired alertness. Breastfeeding mothers should be advised NOT to feed their infant in the lying position (on a bed, sofa or on the floor) as they may fall asleep when breastfeeding and accidentally smother the infant.

Breastfeeding and blood borne viruses

HIV positive mothers should be advised NOT to breastfeed (De Ruiter *et al* 2008). HIV can be transmitted from mother-to-baby *in utero*, during childbirth and through breastfeeding. Breastfeeding can increase the risk of mother-to-child HIV transmission by up to 50% (De Ruiter *et al* 2008, WHO 2008).

Mothers who are hepatitis C positive with chronic infection (i.e. PCR+ve/viraemic) can be encouraged to breastfeed as there is no evidence that breastfeeding increases the risk of mother-to-child transmission of hepatitis C (Scottish Executive 2003, SACDM 2008). The risk of mother-to-child transmission of hepatitis C *in utero* or during childbirth is low – approximately 5% (Department of Health 2007a, NICE 2008a). A woman's hepatitis C status should not influence obstetric management or standard advice regarding breastfeeding (SIGN 2006).

Women who are hepatitis B surface antigen positive ('infectious carriers') can safely breastfeed as soon as their newborn baby has had their first dose of immunoglobulin and first hepatitis B vaccine dose (administered soon after birth).

Infants born to injecting drug users or living in households with injecting drug users should be immunised against hepatitis B.

Weaning advice

Women with problem substance use should seek advice about weaning from their health visitor or GP. Breastfeeding mothers on methadone should be advised to introduce solids into the breastfeeding schedule gradually, reducing the frequency of breast feeds over a number of weeks.

Abrupt cessation of breastfeeding whilst taking methadone (or other opioid substitution therapy and/or benzodiazepines) should be avoided wherever possible, as it may result in the infant showing some signs and symptoms of NAS (Malpas & Darlow 1999). Women who choose to discontinue breastfeeding should develop a plan to wean the baby with their healthcare team (i.e. health visitor and/or GP).

Formula (bottle) feeds are not part of the weaning process. However, if a breastfeeding mother wishes to combine formula feeding with breastfeeding or to switch to formula feeding she should do this gradually, substituting one formula feed for one breast feed per day for several days, allowing her baby and her body to become accustomed to this. A second formula feed can then be introduced for another few days, then a third, fourth etc. Ideally, the weaning process should take several weeks, allowing a slow withdrawal for the baby.

Professionals can also seek advice from *Infant Feeding Advisors* in local maternity services.

Formula (bottle) feeding

Some substance using women may choose to bottle feed rather than breastfeed. Social and cultural beliefs and norms are powerful influences on decision-making about early infant feeding. Parents should be encouraged to breastfeed where possible, and supported to make an informed choice about how to feed their newborn baby. Having made their decision, they should be supported by all professionals involved.

Mothers who choose to bottle feed should be shown how to make up a bottle correctly before they are discharged from hospital, and the community midwife should check to ensure that the advice given has been understood.

Foster care and infant feeding

Some mothers may wish to breastfeed (or continue to breastfeed) their baby even though a decision has been made to place the infant in foster care. These mothers should be supported in their decision to breastfeed as much as possible.

Postnatal care

The care of a pregnant woman who uses drugs or alcohol and the safe delivery of her baby is just the start of care. Continuing support in the postnatal period and for parenthood is essential if the ideal outcome of maintaining a healthy mother and child together, and well functioning family, is to be achieved. Standards for maternity care (RCOG *et al* 2008) recommend that the Department of Health (2009) booklet *'Birth to Five'*, which is a guide to parenthood and the first 5 years of a child's life, should be given to all women within 3 days of birth (if it has not been given antenatally). Practitioners should also refer to the NICE (2006) guidance *Routine postnatal care of women and their babies*.

If the infant is admitted to the neonatal unit for any reason (perhaps because it is preterm, very low birth weight or develops severe drug withdrawal symptoms) then a 'whole family' approach should be adopted – see Department of Health (2009c) *Toolkit for high-quality neonatal services*. Neonatal units should help families cope with the stress, anxiety and altered parenting roles that accompany their baby's condition. This means putting the physical, psychological and social needs of both the baby and their family at the centre of the care process. Family-centred care aims to enhance emotional attachment between the baby and the family in order to improve long-term outcomes for both (Department of Health 2009c).

Before discharge from the postnatal ward or neonatal unit, the family support plan (or child protection plan) should be reviewed. Discharge planning should be multi-disciplinary (organised by the lead professional) and should involve the parents (Department of Health 2009c). Discharge planning is important because it is necessary to make a clear decision about whether the care-giving environment for the baby is safe and nurturing, and the parents understand the developmental needs of the infant and are able to meet those needs.

After discharge from hospital, the baby is cared for at home by the mother and father/family, with advice and support from the community midwife as well as other professionals and agencies involved with the family. The midwife will visit the family at home each day until the baby is 10 days old. Occasionally the midwife may need to continue visiting up until the baby is 28 days old, depending on how well the baby is and how well the mother and father are coping. The health visitor normally visits after day 10 and should liaise with the midwife and GP before visiting the family. The health visitor will be a good source of information and support on parenthood and all aspects of health for the parents and their baby.

When the baby is 6–8 weeks old, the GP or health visitor will organise a postnatal examination of the baby. The woman's physical, emotional and social wellbeing should also be reviewed (NICE 2006). Common maternal health problems include backache, breastfeeding problems, perineal pain, stress incontinence, fatigue, and postnatal depression.

Postnatal care should facilitate the women and her partner to make an effective transition into parenthood. Professionals should give mothers an opportunity to reflect upon their experience of pregnancy and childbirth in the postnatal period as well as an opportunity to discuss the effects of motherhood on their relationships (RCOG *et al* 2008). Fathers should be offered similar support in adjusting to their new role and responsibilities within the family unit (NICE 2006).

Sudden Infant Death Syndrome (SIDS)

Maternal and paternal use of tobacco, alcohol and drugs is associated with an increased risk of Sudden Infant Death Syndrome – 'SIDS' or 'cot death'. All parents who use substances should be given verbal and written advice about how to reduce the risk of cot death. The leaflet *Reducing the risk of cot death* (Department of Health 2009b) is included in the hospital 'discharge pack' and should be discussed with both parents before discharge from hospital.

Risks associated with co-sleeping or bed-sharing

Bed-sharing or co-sleeping, combined with smoking, alcohol and/or other drug use is associated with an increased risk of SIDS (American Academy of Paediatrics 2005). In addition to guidance about Sudden Infant Death Syndrome (SIDS), all parents should be given clear advice about co-sleeping, in line with the Department of Health (2009) guidance. This states that the safest place for a baby to sleep is in a cot in a room with the parents for the first six months. Parents should NEVER share a bed with their baby if either the mother or father:

- smokes (no matter where or when they smoke and even if they do not smoke in bed),
- has recently drunk alcohol,
- has taken medication or drugs which makes them sleep more heavily.

Also advise parents NEVER to sleep with a baby on a sofa or armchair or anywhere else where the parent could roll over whilst asleep and suffocate the baby, or where the baby could get caught between surfaces, or where the baby could roll off and be injured.

The risks associated with co-sleeping are increased if the baby:

● was born preterm (before 37 weeks gestation)
● was low birth weight (less than 2.5kg or 5.51b).

Infant deaths which occur as a result of co-sleeping are extremely distressing for the parents and can be prevented. Ensure that advice about SIDS and co-sleeping is included in the family support plan.

Bonding/attachment

The quality of parent-infant attachment is understood to be a major predictor of long-term outcomes for children, including their social, emotional and behavioural development (NICE 2006). Attachment theory suggests that the development of secure attachment depends upon the care-giver's sensitive responsiveness (or 'attunement') to the infant's cues to provide a context in which the infant's experiences and feelings of security are organised (NICE 2006). The attachment or emotional bond is reciprocal. The infant's behaviour is not only influenced by the care-giver but it may also affect the care-giver's behaviour. More indirect factors may also affect the quality of the development of attachment, including maternal/ paternal personality, level of social support and kinship carer involvement.

Parent-infant attachment can be problematic for substance-using parents for a number of reasons – for example, because of the effects of the parent's substance use on their 'emotional availability', the condition of the baby, a separation from the baby, or all these factors put together. Assessment for emotional attachment should be carried out at each postnatal contact (NICE 2006). Home visits can be used as an opportunity to promote parent-infant attachment, and parents should be encouraged to develop their social networks as this promotes positive parent-infant interaction. Group based parent-training programmes and/or one-to-one interventions designed to promote emotional attachment and improve parenting skills should be offered to parents. Close physical contact through use of soft infant carriers or 'kangaroo techniques', and gentle baby massage, may also promote parent-infant interactions and attachment behaviours (Underdown *et al* 2009, NICE 2006).

Postnatal depression

Mental health problems are very common in people with drug and alcohol problems (Department of Health 2007a). Anxiety, depression, post traumatic stress disorder (PTSD), personality disorder and a history of sexual and/or physical abuse are commonly associated with drug and alcohol dependency. Postnatal depression affects about 10–15% of women who give birth (NICE 2006), and women substance users may be more at risk of postnatal depression because of previous or existing mental health issues, social isolation and poor partner support. Identifying and supporting women at risk of postnatal depression is very important. Untreated postnatal depression is associated with detrimental effects on parent-infant interactions and infant development (particularly cognitive and emotional disturbance). Children of depressed mothers are more likely to suffer from mental health problems as adolescents and adults and access child and adolescent mental health services more (NICE 2006). Postnatal depression is normally assessed around 10–14 days after birth, using a screening tool such as the *Edinburgh Postnatal Depression Score* (EPDS). Health visitors and GPs are trained to use these tools to improve the care of women at risk.

Puerperal psychosis, the most severe form of postpartum psychiatric illness, affects 1–2 women per thousand (SIGN 2002). It usually presents in the early postpartum period, within the first month, and is largely affective in nature (i.e. severe disorder of mood).

Staff should make themselves familiar with the following helpful clinical guidelines:
- *Postnatal Depression and Puerperal Psychosis* (SIGN 2002)
- *Antenatal and postnatal mental health: clinical management and service guidance* (NICE 2007a)

Further good practice guidance on working with parents with mental health problems and their children includes:
- *Think child, think parent, think family: a guide to parental mental health and child welfare* (SCIE 2009).

Risk of relapse

In the postnatal period, increased drug and alcohol use is common. For mothers who have managed to reduce their intake during pregnancy or even come off drugs or alcohol, the risk of relapse to former levels of drinking or drug taking is high. There are a number of reasons for this, including:

- wanting to celebrate
- feeling that it's now OK to use again
- relief at having a 'normal' baby
- 'baby blues' or postnatal depression
- the stress of caring for a newborn baby (perhaps with NAS)
- poor support from partner, family or friends
- anxieties about parenthood
- stress in relation to child protection procedures and interventions.

It is important for professionals to acknowledge that relapse is common. Re-assessment of substance use and careful drug/alcohol management is essential at this time, along with support to remain stable and to prevent relapse and the risk of accidental drug overdose.

Ensuring the woman and her partner, if appropriate, is engaged with a specialist drug/alcohol agency that can provide a relapse prevention service and other psychosocial interventions (NICE 2007c) may be an important part of the postnatal family support plan.

Relapse prevention work (Witkiewitz & Marlatt 2004) can include:

- helping parents understand relapse as a process and as an event.
- raising awareness of 'high-risk' situations and factors that might lead to relapse.
- exploring how to anticipate, avoid or cope with high-risk situations.
- acquisition of skills (cognitive and behavioural) to implement relapse prevention strategies.
- anxiety and stress management education.
- confidence building and improving self-efficacy.
- strengthening existing positive coping strategies and other personal attributes.
- life/social skills education (e.g. assertiveness, resistance and dissuasion skills, alternative activities to drug/alcohol use).
- introduction to recovery-orientated peer support groups or networks.
- involvement of close family and friends to support a 'community reinforcement approach' (Meyers et al 2005).

Safe storage of drugs and alcohol in the home

The arrival of a new baby is a good opportunity to raise the subject of safety issues within the home and to discuss the safe storage of drugs and alcohol, even if this has been done before. A number of infants and children in the UK have died or nearly died as a result of adults exposing them to dangerous drugs. Over half of all poisoning cases in children are caused by them swallowing medication or other substances obtained within the home environment (HM Government 2011).

All parents with problem substance use should be told how to store dangerous substances safely so they are 'out of sight' and 'out of reach' of children. Parents should be advised that only a tiny amount of methadone can kill a child and that immediate medical attention must be sought if a child accidentally swallows any substance. An information leaflet for parents '*Keeping children safe from alcohol and drugs in the home*' (see appendix 2) contains further advice about this subject and can be given to mothers and fathers.

Assessing parenting capacity and child care risk during pregnancy

Many pregnant women who have problem substance use worry that they will be referred to social services or their baby will be taken into care purely because they use drugs or alcohol. Raising this subject early and discussing their concerns openly will foster a more trusting relationship and will help them overcome their fears (NICE 2010a). It is important to reassure women that problem substance use, *in itself*, is not sufficient reason to assume inadequate parenting or child care. They need to know, however, that if there are specific concerns about the safety or welfare of the child then social work may need to do an assessment and get involved, but that this policy is the same for everyone, whether or not they use alcohol or drugs. This advice is included in the information leaflet *Pregnant... and using drugs and alcohol* (see appendix 4).

Many different factors affect the health and development of children. Parental drug and alcohol use is just one factor. Research evidence does not support the assumption that parental substance use will automatically lead to child neglect or abuse (Scottish Executive 2003, Kroll & Taylor 2003, Templeton *et al* 2007). However, parenting capacity is often compromised and child protection involvement is common in families where maternal or paternal substance use is problematic, usually on account of neglect (ACMD 2003, Kroll & Taylor 2003, Barnard & McKeganey 2004, Forrester 2007, Street *et al* 2008, Cleaver *et al* 2010). Infants, in particular, are vulnerable to the effects of physical and emotional neglect which can have damaging effects on their long term development (ACMD 2003).

It is important to remember that becoming 'drug free' should not be a requirement for parents to keep their children living with them or to be considered a 'good enough' parent. Parents who stop using drugs or control their drug or alcohol intake are not necessarily better or safer parents. Some parents will have poor parenting capacity for reasons other than their substance use as many risk factors also occur in non-substance-using families (Sidebotham 2001, Scottish Executive 2003, Templeton *et al* 2007, Cleaver *et al* 2010). However, fluctuating drug or alcohol use and a disorganised lifestyle may affect child safety and the child's health and development in a number of ways and is always a factor to be considered.

Childcare problems that have been associated with parental problem substance use (ACMD 2003, Kroll & Taylor 2003, Cleaver *et al* 2010) include:

- Inconsistent caring
- Inadequate supervision
- Lack of stimulation
- Inadequate and unsafe accommodation
- Social isolation and stigma
- Exposure to violence and criminal behaviour
- Emotional or physical neglect or abuse.

Resulting in...

- Failure to thrive
- Accidental injury
- Emotional difficulties
- Behavioural difficulties
- Poor social development
- Poor cognitive development and educational attainment.

Professionals who are involved with children and families need to remember that good inter-agency communication and collaboration is essential. It is important to obtain consent from the parents early to share information with other professionals and agencies. No professional, however, can guarantee absolute confidentiality as both statute and common law accepts that information may be shared in certain circumstances.

Child care risk assessment should cover issues such as parenting skills, child safety, as well as the physical, cognitive, emotional and social development of children. Drug and alcohol specialist workers that lack child care and parenting expertise should consult with and involve other professionals and agencies who do have this expertise. Likewise, children's services should consult with alcohol and drug specialists to consider the nature and extent of the parent's substance use and how this impacts, or is likely to impact, on the child's wellbeing. Guidance on joint working between drug and alcohol treatment services and children and family services is available – see DCSF/Department of Health/NTA (2009). Scottish Executive (2003) guidance '*Getting Our Priorities Right: Good practice Guidance for working with Children and Families affected by Substance Misuse*', also includes a helpful checklist for collating information on problem substance use and its impact on parenting (download from www.scotland.gov.uk).

Safeguarding children

The welfare of the child is the paramount consideration. All professionals working with pregnant women and families affected by problem substance use should make themselves familiar with their local Inter-agency Child Protection Procedures.

The assessment process may highlight concerns because the woman or her partner:
- has multiple or complex social problems
- has a disorganised lifestyle which means they repeatedly fail to attend antenatal appointments
- attends appointments but are repeatedly intoxicated or incapacitated from the effects of alcohol or drugs
- has serious mental health problems
- has multiple or serious criminal convictions
- has an inappropriate home environment which could be unsafe for a baby
- lacks the necessary material possessions for a baby
- has been previously referred to social work regarding their parenting capacity
- has existing children living with kinship carers
- has existing children on the child protection register
- has had previous children accommodated by the local authority
- has had previous children adopted
- discloses domestic abuse
- is socially isolated with no social support network.

Professionals who have concerns could consider taking one or more of the following actions:
- Refer to a non-statutory service that works with children and families affected by problem substance use. Substance-using parents see non-statutory services as more acceptable and less 'stigmatising' and threatening than social services. Practitioners who work in these services can offer intensive parenting support.
- Discuss your concerns with the midwife, health visitor or general practitioner
- Contact your designated senior staff member with responsibility for child protection to discuss your concerns
- Contact your local duty social work service (Children and Families Team) to discuss your concerns and to seek their advice.
- Encourage the woman and her partner to approach social services themselves for help and advice.

- Make a referral to Children and Families social work service and discuss this action with the parents.

If there is a significant risk of harm to the baby's health and development then professionals should take action and refer to social services. Harm may result from maltreatment or the absence of adequate care. Safeguarding children is an interagency responsibility, but social work has a statutory responsibility to assess risk and ensure that child protection plans are in place if necessary. The social work assessment, while acknowledging the needs and the rights of the parents, will focus primarily on the needs and welfare of the child. In some situations there will be conflict between the needs and wishes of the parents and the welfare of the child.

Any referral or discussion with social services should be handled sensitively. It is important to stress to the woman and her partner that social work involvement is often positive and helpful. Whenever possible, social work has a duty to promote children's upbringing by their families. Compulsory and permanent removal of children from their families is rare, even when agencies are concerned about a child's welfare (Scottish Executive 2003).

On occasion, social services will be sufficiently concerned about the future risk to an unborn child to warrant the implementation of child protection procedures and the calling of a child protection case conference to consider the need for a child protection plan. If a child protection case conference is called, ideally it should be held around 28 weeks gestation so that services can be put in place in time for the birth of the baby.

Early intervention strategies

For families who are 'of concern' but not formally 'at risk', professionals should take the opportunity to engage with the parents and intervene early. A range of interventions can be helpful for vulnerable children and families (Cabinet Office 2008). These include offering parenting support by:
- Offering emotional support and an opportunity to talk about any stresses or worries
- Discussing parenting roles and responsibilities
- Developing the parents' existing skills, attributes and resources
- Promoting a safer and more stable lifestyle
- Teaching strategies to develop good parent/infant attachment
- Offering or arranging practical support to the family

- Teaching good play techniques and parent/child activities
- Discussing strategies for managing their children's behaviour
- Teaching parents how to gauge the developmental needs of their children
- Engaging families in activities where they can experience positive role modelling
- Helping parents develop family routines, rules and boundaries with their children.

Promoting recovery, resilience and protective factors

The majority of pregnant women and parents with substance use problems can provide good parenting and child care if given the right support at the right time. An 'ecological approach' and strengths-based models of intervention are known to be most effective (Sidebotham 2001, Velleman & Templeton 2007, Cabinet Office 2008). This involves taking a holistic approach and identifying strengths and stressors in the individual, the family and the environment, and then assisting to promote the strengths and decrease the stressors (Cabinet Office 2008). This approach involves promoting resilience, strengthening protective factors, and taking a wider social inclusion perspective. Good parenting is as much a feature of parent's neighbourhood, social networks and social environment as it is an individual attribute. Recent research highlights the importance of looking at the family as a whole (Cabinet Office 2008), and focusing on building positive supportive relationships and social networks – 'social capital' (Velleman & Templeton 2007). Both adult and children's services have a role to play in helping to build family resources, resilience, stability and social integration.

Professionals who provide care to pregnant women and their partners can ensure that 'protective factors' are promoted by routinely discussing the following topics both before and after the baby is born:
- The importance of providing for all the child's basic needs... food, clothes, warmth, personal hygiene, comfort, safety, stimulation, age-appropriate activities etc.
- The importance of attending child health appointments with the GP, health visitor (public health nurse), and community paediatrician.
- The importance of providing appropriate supervision for their children – periods of intoxication and withdrawal may be a time when adequate supervision cannot be provided and parents will need to ensure that another responsible adult is available in these situations.

- The importance of establishing and maintaining routines and making the home safe and secure for the child.
- The importance of seeking support from family and friends and professionals in times of stress.
- Outlining potential problems such as a chaotic lifestyle, other substance-using friends and households, procurement of drugs, violence in the home or in the neighbourhood, drug dealing, and offending behaviour which may put the child at risk.
- Discussing safe storage of alcohol and drugs in the home, including safe storage of medication, safe storage and disposal of injecting equipment, risks of ingestion of drugs and overdose, how to deal with medical emergencies etc.
- Promoting regular contact and involvement with non drug-using friends and family.

A wider social inclusion perspective might include helping parents with budgeting and financial problems, housing, legal problems, training, education and employment. It is hard for parents to concentrate on their recovery if they are worried about keeping a roof over their head, or the threat of imprisonment, or providing a meal for their children. A holistic package of support that takes into account the wider needs of the family is required.

Finally, it is important to remember that pregnancy is a special event in the life of a woman with substance use problems and provides professionals with an opportunity to offer treatment and care that might not otherwise be accepted. The philosophy of approach and principles of management should be broadly the same as for any other pregnant woman with special circumstances and additional needs. Research on fathers and fatherhood over the past few decades has also highlighted the needs of fathers in relation to parenting, child care and family life (Lewis & Lamb 2007). The inclusion of fathers in pregnancy, parenting and child welfare services is now understood to be essential, not optional, and will help to achieve a 'whole family' approach.

Further help, information, useful addresses and websites

Royal College of Obstetricians and Gynaecologists (RCOG)
www.rcog.org.uk

Royal College of Midwives (RCM)
www.rcm.org.uk

Royal College of Nurses (RCN)
www.rcn.org.uk

Royal College of General Practitioners (RCGP)
www.rcgp.org.uk
including 'Emma's Diary', support site for women who are pregnant
www.emmasdiary.co.uk

Royal College of Paediatrics and Child Health (RCPCH)
www.rcpch.ac.uk

Royal College of Psychiatrists (RCPsych)
www.rcpsych.ac.uk

British Association of Social Workers (BASW)
www.basw.co.uk

National Institute for Health and Clinical Excellence (NICE)
www.nice.org.uk

Scottish Intercollegiate Guidelines Network (SIGN)
www.sign.ac.uk

Family Planning Association (FPA)
Helpline 0845 122 8690
www.fpa.org.uk

National Childbirth Trust (NCT)
Pregnancy and birth helpline 0300 330 0772
Breastfeeding helpline 0300 330 0771

Postnatal helpline 0300 330 0773
www.nct.org.uk

Fatherhood Institute
www.fatherhoodinstitute.org

'The Pregnancy Book'
Department of Health (England, Wales, Northern Ireland) updated June 2010
www.dh.gov.uk/en/Publicationsandstatistics/Publications/
PublicationsPolicyAndGuidance/DH_107302

'Ready, Steady, Baby! A Guide to Pregnancy, Birth and Early Parenthood'
NHS Health Scotland
www.readysteadybaby.org.uk

Smoking, alcohol and drug specific information

SmokeFree (Department of Health website)
Smokeline (NHS free helpline) 0800 022 4332
www.smokefree.nhs.uk

CanStopSmoking (NHS Scotland)
Smokeline (NHS Scotland free helpline) 0800 84 8484
www.canstopsmoking.com

Action on Smoking and Health (ASH)
www.ash.org.uk

ASH Scotland
www.ashscotland.org.uk

Drinkline – UK helpline 0800 917 8282

Alcohol Concern
www.alcoholconcern.org.uk

Alcohol Focus Scotland
www.alcohol-focus-scotland.org.uk

Alcoholics Anonymous (UK)
National helpline 0845 769 7555
www.alcoholics-anonymous.org.uk

National Organisation on Fetal Alcohol Syndrome (UK)
www.nofas-uk.org

FRANK – The UK National Drugs Helpline
Tel. 0800 77 66 00 (24 hours a day)
www.talktofrank.com

National Treatment Agency for Substance Misuse (NTA)
www.nta.nhs.uk

DrugScope
www.drugscope.org.uk

Scottish Drugs Forum (SDF)
www.sdf.org.uk

UK Narcotics Anonymous
National helpline 0300 999 1212
www.ukna.org

Blood borne viruses and sexual health

British HIV Association (BHIVA)
www.bhiva.org

Children's HIV Association (CHIVA)
www.chiva.org.uk

British Association for Sexual Health and HIV (BASHH)
www.bashh.org

British Liver Trust
Helpline 0800 652 7330
www.britishlivertrust.org.uk

The Hepatitis C Trust
Helpline 0845 223 4424
www.hepctrust.org.uk

Children's Liver Disease Foundation
www.childliverdisease.org

Other useful resources

Women's Aid
National Domestic Violence helpline 0808 2000 247
www.womensaid.org.uk

Scottish Women's Aid
Domestic Abuse helpline (Scotland) 0800 027 1234
www.scottishwomensaid.org.uk

National Society for the Prevention of Cruelty to Children (NSPCC)
Including National Child Protection helpline 0808 800 5000
www.nspcc.org.uk

Family and Parenting Institute
www.familyandparenting.org

Evidence Based Practice parenting programmes
www.commissioningtoolkit.org

Policy Research Bureau – parenting database
www.prb.org.uk/wwiparenting

Every Child Matters – information and guidance
www.education.gov.uk (undertake a search)

Common Assessment Framework (CAF) – information and guidance
www.education.gov.uk (undertake a search)

Getting it right for every child (GIRFEC) – information and guidance
www.scotland.gov.uk/Topics/People/Young-People/childrensservices/girfec

Think Family Toolkit – 'Improving support for families at risk' guidance
http://publications.education.gov.uk/default.aspx?PageFunction=productdetails&
PageMode=publications&ProductId=DCSF-00685–2009&

Glossary

Amniotic fluid	Fluid that surrounds the baby in the uterus (sometimes called liquor – pronounced lye-kwor).
Antenatal	Before the birth.
Antenatal care	Care provided by professionals during pregnancy in order to detect, predict, prevent and manage problems in the woman or her unborn child.
APGAR score	Score measured at birth by observations of the babies health e.g. colour, tone, heart rate etc.
Benzodiazepines	A class of drugs previously called 'minor tranquillisers' which reduce anxiety and have a sedative effect.
Binge drinking	Excessive amount of alcohol taken on any one occasion, usually twice the recommended daily amount (i.e. 6 units or more for women).
Bio-physical profile assessment	Use of ultrasound scanning to assess fetal wellbeing.
Birth plan	A written record of a woman's preferences for her care during pregnancy, labour and childbirth.
Booking	The appointment where the mother enters the maternity care pathway, characterised by information giving and detailed history taking, routine antenatal screening and care planning – normally undertaken by a community midwife.
Brief intervention	Usually consists of a brief assessment of substance use, information and advice on the risks associated with substance use and how to reduce these risks, and details of local services and other helpful resources.

Caesarean Section	An operation where the baby is delivered through an incision through the abdomen and uterus.
Care Pathways	Structured multidisciplinary care plans which detail essential steps in the treatment and care of patients with a specific illness or condition.
Child's Plan	A co-ordinated structured plan that agrees desired outcomes for a child, and the methods of achieving change. It includes timescales, responsibilities, any services that need to be provided in order to meet the child's needs, a contingency plan, and records the partners/service providers involved in the plan.
Child Protection Case Conference	A multi-disciplinary meeting convened by social work professionals to assess the level of risk to children and to decide on what action needs to be taken, if any.
CNS depressant	A drug which acts on the central nervous system to suppress neural activity in the brain e.g. opioids and benzodiazepines.
CNS stimulant	A drug which acts on the central nervous system to increase neural activity in the brain e.g. amphetamines, cocaine, nicotine.
Conception	The act of becoming pregnant.
Concern	A concern is something which affects or has the potential to affect the safety, wellbeing or potential of a child. It may relate to a single event or observation, a series of events, an attribute of the child or someone associated with them, or a feature of the child's care-giving environment.
Congenital abnormalities	An anomaly present at birth.

Continuity of care	A situation where all professionals involved in delivery of care share common ways of working and a common philosophy so that the woman does not experience conflicting experience or advice.
Detoxification	Process by which a user withdraws from the effects of alcohol or drugs over a short period of time (i.e. 1 to 4 weeks), usually managed with medication.
Deprivation category	The Carstairs and Morris index is composed of 4 indicators judged to represent material disadvantage in the population. These include: overcrowding, male unemployment, social class 4 or 5 and no car.
Drug/Alcohol Dependence	A syndrome characterised by a cluster of signs and symptoms including physical dependence (e.g. tolerance and withdrawal) and psychological dependence (e.g. compulsion, avoidance behaviour, disregard for harm).
Drug/Alcohol related problem	Refers to a whole spectrum of harm (physical, psychological, social) associated with substance use.
Early intervention	Taking action to assess need/risk to children/unborn children and to provide support/services early to a family in order to prevent escalation and/or deterioration.
Ectopic pregnancy	A pregnancy that develops somewhere other than the uterus, usually in the fallopian tube – the pregnancy cannot be allowed to continue as it is dangerous.
EDD	Expected date of delivery – when the baby is due (sometimes called EDC – expected date of confinement).
Episiotomy	A cut made in the perineum (the area between the vagina and anus) to allow the baby to be born more quickly and to prevent tearing.

Family Support Plan	A Family Support Plan (FSP) is a tool to document and guide the care plan process for children and families. The FSP contains information about the services necessary to facilitate a child's development and enhance the family's capacity to facilitate the child's development. Through the FSP process, family members and service providers work as a team to plan, implement, and evaluate services tailored to the family's unique needs, concerns, priorities, and resources.
Fetal	Of the fetus or unborn child.
General practitioners (GPs)	Are doctors who have responsibility for providing general medical care to the whole family and in most circumstances will confirm the pregnancy. GPs are experienced in caring for pregnant women and work closely with community midwives. Many jointly manage antenatal care in Primary Care Health Centres. They also work closely with obstetricians and midwives to providing care to women with 'high risk' pregnancies. GPs provide postnatal care to both mother and baby and work closely with health visitors to monitor and improve the health and development of children. In many areas, people with a drug dependency who are on substitute drugs (e.g. methadone) are managed by their GP and attend primary care for their prescription.
Gestation	Age of fetus since conception.
Gravid	Pregnant.

Health visitors/ public health nurses	Are nurses who specialise in family and public health and are part of the primary care team. They work alongside midwives to provide parent education and support during and after pregnancy. At the point when midwifery care ends (normally 10 days after birth) the health visitor takes responsibility for the mother, baby and family and will visit in the immediate postnatal period, then follow-up the child until the child starts school. Health visitors play a key role in supporting families with breastfeeding, postnatal depression, diet, exercise, child health and development, disease prevention, parenting, behaviour management, social and emotional issues. Health visitors visit pregnant women before they give birth and get involved in their care at an early stage.
'High Risk' pregnancy	Pregnancy with increased likelihood of complications, usually managed by an obstetrician.
Harmful drinking	Levels of drinking which cause physical or psychological harm.
Infant	A child in the first year of life.
Injecting paraphernalia	All the equipment used for injecting drugs e.g. spoon, filter, cup, needle, syringe etc.
Intoxication	A state where the individual has drunk or taken drugs sufficient to significantly impair functions such as speech, thinking, or ability to walk or drive.
Intrapartum care	Care provided during labour and childbirth.
Intrauterine growth restriction (IUGR)	Restricted fetal growth. Previously known as intrauterine growth retardation.
In-utero	In the uterus or womb, unborn.

Lead professional	A professional involved with the family who is responsible for ensuring that the family has access to care from other professionals as appropriate, and who will often provide a substantial part of the care personally.
'Low risk' pregnancy	Normal pregnancy with few anticipated complications, usually managed by a midwife.
Midwifery team	A small team of midwives (normally based in the community) who share responsibility for care during pregnancy, childbirth and the postnatal period.
Midwives	Are specially trained in pregnancy, childbirth and postnatal care, and usually manage 'low risk' pregnancies independently. The midwife undertakes a continuous risk assessment throughout pregnancy and refers to other appropriate medical professionals if they detect deviations from the norm. They also have a significant role in health education and in supporting parents in the transition to parenthood. All pregnant women are allocated a named midwife at booking. This will normally be a midwife attached to their GP surgery.
Meta-analysis	Results from a collection of independent studies (investigating the same phenomenon) which are pooled using statistical techniques to synthesise the findings into one estimate.
Multigravida/ Multiparous	A woman who has been pregnant before/who has carried more than one pregnancy to a viable stage.
Named professional	A practitioner who has responsibility for ensuring that an adult/child's needs are addressed in health and social care services. Sometimes called 'key worker'.
NAS	Neonatal Abstinence Syndrome.
Neonatal Abstinence Syndrome (NAS)	A group of drug withdrawal symptoms affecting newborn infants whose mother has been using certain substances, usually opiates and benzodiazepines.

Neonatal period	First 28 days of a baby's life.
Neonate	A newborn infant.
Neonatologists and paediatricians	Are doctors who have the responsibility for looking after the medical needs of babies, including preterm infants, babies who are ill (for instance with Neonatal Abstinence Syndrome), and babies with congenital abnormalities. They work closely with obstetricians, midwives, neonatal nurses and health visitors to plan and provide care for infants in partnership with the parents. Neonates who are ill are normally cared for in the Neonatal Unit (NNU) or Special Care Baby Unit (SCBU).
Nulliparous	A woman who has not given birth to a viable infant.
Obstetric	The branch of medicine and surgery that deals with pregnancy and childbirth.
Obstetricians and gynaecologists	Are doctors who are experts in all aspects of pregnancy and childbirth. Obstetricians have expertise in treating complications of pregnancy and childbirth and offer specialist advice, screening and treatment. Obstetricians manage 'high risk' pregnancies, usually with midwifery and GP support.
Opiates	Drugs derived from the opium poppy e.g. heroin, morphine, codeine.
Opioids	Includes both opiates and their synthetic analogues e.g. methadone, dihydrocodeine, pethidine.
Parity	The number of maternities to a woman (children born live or stillbirth after 24 weeks gestation).
Parous	A woman who has given birth to at least one viable offspring (usually more than 24 weeks gestation).

Pharmacists	Work in partnership with patients, doctors and other health care professionals to ensure medicines are used safely and to best effect. Many community pharmacists are in frequent contact with pregnant women who use substances, so can provide support and healthcare advice. Pharmacists provide a wide range of services including: smoking cessation, dispensing of 'substitute' prescriptions, supervised self-administration of methadone, needle exchange schemes, and general health promotion advice.
Placenta praevia	When the placenta is low down, sometimes covering the cervix, blocking the baby's exit, which would require a caesarean section.
Postnatal	After the birth.
Postpartum care	Care provided in the period following delivery.
Polydrug use	The use of more than one drug at a time.
Preterm	A baby born before 37 weeks gestation (a 'full-term' pregnancy lasts 40 weeks).
Primigravida/ primipara	A woman pregnant for the first time – sometimes called 'prim'.
Problem drug/ alcohol use	Tends to refer to drug use (dependent or recreational) which causes health, social, financial, or legal problems.
Recreational drug use	The occasional use of drugs for pleasure or leisure.
Reproductive health	Health of the organs involved in the process of conception, pregnancy and childbirth.
Resuscitation	Revival of someone who is in cardiac or respiratory failure or shock.
Rooming in	Practice of ensuring mother and baby stay together 24 hours a day after delivery – this helps with feeding and bonding and it reduces the risk of infection.

Screening	Mass examination of the population to detect specific illnesses or conditions.
Shared care	An agreed arrangement between a GP and an obstetrician/midwife/paediatrician/or other health specialist over care for a woman.
Skin-to-skin contact	Where the baby is placed directly onto the mothers'/parents' bare skin (usually chest).
Social inclusion	Ensuring that everyone regardless of sex, wealth, race, religion, age, lifestyle and geographical position has the opportunity to live full and active lives free from injustice, discrimination and poverty.
Stillbirth	Baby born dead after 24 completed weeks of pregnancy. Stillbirths must be registered and the cause of death established before a certificate of stillbirth can be issued and a burial take place.
Substance misuse/abuse	Taken to mean the use of drugs or alcohol in a socially unacceptable and harmful way.
Systematic review	A review where evidence from research studies has been identified, appraised and synthesised in a methodical way according to predetermined criteria.
Teratogenic	Causing fetal malformations or congenital birth defects.
Term	40 weeks gestation or thereabouts from the first day of the last menstrual period.
Tolerance	Higher doses of drug are needed to maintain the same effect.
Trimester	Each period of three months in pregnancy (1st, 2nd and 3rd trimesters).
Ultrasound scan	Image created by use of sound waves, which can confirm pregnancy and determine fetal size and wellbeing.
Umbilical artery Doppler	Is a fetal monitoring assessment test.

Vertical transmission	Transmission from mother to baby either in utero, during childbirth or through breastfeeding.
Viral load	The amount of virus circulating in the blood.
Volatile substances	Refers to solvents and inhalants including aerosols.
Withdrawal	The body's reaction to the sudden absence of alcohol or a drug to which it has adapted.

References

Aaron S, *et al* (2008) Intranasal transmission of hepatitis C virus: virological and clinical evidence, *Clinical Infectious Diseases*, 4, 7, 931–934.

Aase JM, *et al* (1970) Children of mothers who took LSD in pregnancy, *Lancet*, 11, 100–101.

Abdel-Latif ME, *et al* (2006) Effects of breast milk on the severity and outcome of neonatal abstinence syndrome among infants of drug-dependent mothers, *Pediatrics*, 117, 6, 1163–1169.

Abel EL. (1998) *Fetal Alcohol Syndrome*, Plenum Press, New York.

ACMD (2003) *Hidden Harm: responding to the needs of children of problem drug users, The report of an Inquiry by the Advisory Council on the Misuse of Drugs*, London, Home Office.

ACOG (2008) *At-risk drinking and illicit drug use: ethical issues in obstetric and gynaecologic practice. ACOG Committee Opinion, NO.422*, American College of Obstetricians and Gynecologists.

Addis A. *et al* (2001) Fetal effects of cocaine: an updated meta-analysis. *Reproductive Toxicology*, 15, 341–369.

Alcohol and Pregnancy Project (2009) *Alcohol and Pregnancy and Fetal Alcohol Spectrum Disorder: a Resource for Health Professionals (1st revision)*. Perth, Telethon Institute for Child Health Research.

Almario CV. *et al* (2009) Risk factors for preterm birth among opiate-addicted gravid women in a methadone treatment program. *American Journal of Obstetrics and Gynecology*, 201, 326–326.e6.

American Academy of Pediatrics (1998) Neonatal drug withdrawal, *Pediatrics*, 101, 6, 1079–1086.

American Academy of Pediatrics (2005) The changing concept of Sudden Infant Death Syndrome: diagnostic coding shifts, controversies regarding the sleeping environment, and new variables to consider in reducing risk, Task Force on Sudden Infant Death Syndrome, *Pediatrics*, 116, 1245–1255.

Ashley SJ, & Little RE. (1990) Maternal marijuana use during lactation and infant development at one year, *Neurotoxicology and Teratology*, 12, 2, 161–168.

Astley SJ. (2004) *Diagnostic Guide for Fetal Alcohol Spectrum Disorders: The 4-Digit Diagnostic Code.* Seattle: University of Washington.

Baldacchino A., Riglietta M., & Corkery J. Eds. (2003) *Maternal health and drug abuse: Perspectives across Europe*, European Collaborating Centres in Addiction Studies, Monograph Series NO.3, ECCAS, Denmark.

Babor TF, *et al* (2001) *AUDIT the alcohol use disorders identification test: guidelines for use in primary care*, 2nd Edition, Geneva, Department of Mental Health and Substance Dependence, World Health Organisation.

Babor TF, & Higgins-Biddle JC. (2001) *Brief intervention for hazardous and harmful drinking: a manual for use in primary care*, Geneva, Department of Mental Health and Substance Dependence, World Health Organisation.

Barnard M, & McKeganey N. (2004) The impact of parental problem drug use on children: what is the problem and what can be done to help? *Addiction.* 99: 552–9.

Barnish M. (2004) *Domestic violence: a literature review*, HM Inspectorate of Probation, London, Home Office.

Bauer CR, *et al* (2005) Acute neonatal effects of cocaine exposure during pregnancy. *Archives Paediatric Adolescent Medicine*, 159, 824–834.

Begg EJ, et al. (2001) Distribution of R- and S-methadone into human milk during multiple, medium and high oral dosing, *British Journal of Clinical Pharmacology*, 52, 681 –685.

Bell J, & Harvey-Dodds L. (2008) Pregnancy and injecting drug use, *British Medical Journal*, 7, 336, 1303–1305.

Berghella V, *et al* (2003) Maternal methadone dose and neonatal withdrawal. *American Journal of Obstetrics and Gynaecology*, 189, 2, 312–317.

Best D, & Abdulrahim D. (2005) *Women in drug treatment services: Research briefing: 6*, London, National Treatment Agency.

Binder T. & Vavinkova B. (2008) Prospective randomised comparative study of the effect of buprenorphine, methadone and heroin on the course of pregnancy, birthweight of newborns, early postpartum adaptation and course of the neonatal abstinence syndrome (NAS) in women followed up in the outpatient department, *Neuroendocrinology Letters*, 29, 1, 80–86.

Blair PS, et al. (1999) Babies sleeping with parents: case-control study of factors influencing the risk of sudden infant death syndrome, *British Medical Journal*, 319, 7223, 1457–1462.

Blinick G, et al. (1975) Methadone assays in pregnant women and progeny. *American Journal of Obstetrics and Gynecology*. 121, 617–621.

BMA (2007a) *Fetal alcohol spectrum disorders: a guide for healthcare professionals*, London, British Medical Association.

BMA (2007b) *Domestic abuse: a report from the BMA Board of Science*, London, British Medical Association.

BHIVA, BASHH, BIS (2008) *UK National Guidelines for HIV Testing 2008*, British HIV Association, British Association of Sexual Health and HIV, British Infection Society. www.bhiva.org

BHIVA/CHIVA (2008) *Guidelines for the management of HIV infection in pregnant women*, British HIV Association & Children's HIV Association. www.bhiva.org

Bradley KA, *et al* (1998) Alcohol Screening questionnaires in women: A Critical Review, *JAMA*, 280, 2, p166–71.

Brandon M, et al. (2008) *Analysing child deaths and serious injury through abuse and neglect: what can we learn? A biennial analysis of serious case reviews 2003–2005: Research Report DCSF-RR023*. London, Department for Children, Schools and Families.

Brandon M, *et al* (2009) *Understanding Serious Case Reviews and their Impact: A Biennial Analysis of Serious Case Reviews 2005–2007*. London: Department for Children Schools and Families.

Broekhuizen FF, *et al* (1992) Drug use or inadequate prenatal care? Adverse pregnancy outcome in an urban setting, *American Journal of Obstetrics & Gynecology*, 166, 1747–1756.

Brook G, *et al* (2010) British HIV Association guidelines for the management of co-infection with HIV-1 and hepatitis B or C virus 2010, *HIV Medicine*, 11, 1–30.

Burns C, *et al* (1996) The health and development of children whose mothers are on methadone maintenance. *Child Abuse Review*, 5, 113–122.

Cabinet Office (2008a) *Think Family: a literature review of whole family approaches*, London, Social Exclusion Task Force, Cabinet Office.

Cabinet Office (2008b) *Think Family: improving the life chances of families at risk*, London, Social Exclusion Task Force, Cabinet Office.

Cairns PA. (2001) Drug misuse: conception into childhood, *Current Paediatrics*, 11, 475–479.

CEMACH (2007) *Saving mothers' lives: reviewing maternal deaths to make motherhood safer 2003–2005*. London, Confidential Enquiry Maternal and Child Health.

Center for Substance Abuse Treatment (2004) *Clinical guidelines for the use of buprenorphine in the treatment of opioid addiction: A treatment improvement protocol (TIP) 40*. Rockville, U.S. Department of Health and Human Services: Substance Abuse and Mental Health Services Administration.

Chang G., *et al* (1999) Brief intervention for alcohol use in pregnancy: A randomised trial, *Addiction*, 94, 10, 1499–1508.

Chang G, *et al* (2006) Identifying risk drinking in expectant fathers. *Birth: Issues in Perinatal Care*, 33, 2, 110–116.

Choo RE. *et al* (2004) Neonatal Abstinence Syndrome in methadone-exposed infants is altered by level of prenatal tobacco exposure. *Drug and Alcohol Dependence*, 75, 253–260.

Cleaver H. *et al* (2010) *Children's Needs – Parenting Capacity: The impact of parental mental illness, learning disability, problem alcohol and drug use, and domestic violence on children's safety and development.* 2nd Edition. London: The Stationery Office.

Coghlan D, *et al* (1999) Neonatal Abstinence Syndrome, *Irish Medical Journal*, 92, 1.

Craig M. (2001) Substance misuse in pregnancy, *Current Obstetrics & Gynaecology*, 11, 365–371.

Daniel B. & Taylor J. (2001) *Engaging with fathers*, London, Jessica Kingsley.

Dashe JS, *et al* (2002) Relationship between maternal methadone dosage and neonatal withdrawal, *Obstetrics & Gynecology*, 100, 6, 1244–1249.

Day E. & George S. (2005) Management of drug misuse in pregnancy, *Advances in Psychiatric Treatment*, 11, 253–261.

Department of Health (2000) *Framework for the assessment of children in need and their families*, London, HMSO.

Department of Health (2003) *Infant feeding recommendation*, London, Department of Health.

Department of Health (2004a) *Maternity Standard, National Service Framework for Children, Young People and Maternity Services*, Change for Children – Every Child Matters, London, Department of Health.

Department of Health (2004b) *Good practice and innovation in breastfeeding*, London, Department of Health.

Department of Health (2005) *Responding to domestic abuse: a handbook for health professionals*, London, Department of Health.

Department of Health (2007a) *Drug Misuse and dependence: UK guidelines on clinical management*, London, Department of Health (England) and the devolved administrations.

Department of Health (2007b) *Maternity Matters: choice, access and continuity of care in a safe service*, London, Department of Health.

Department of Health (2009a) *The pregnancy book*, London, Department of Health.

Department of Health (2009b) *Improving safety, Reducing harm: Children, young people and domestic violence: A practical toolkit for front-line practitioners*. London, Department of Health.

Department of Health (2009c) *Toolkit for high quality neonatal services*, London, Department of Health.

Department of Health (2009d) *Reducing the risk of cot death,* London, Department of Health.

De Ruiter A, *et al* (2008) British HIV Association and Children's HIV Association guidelines for the management of HIV infection in pregnant women 2008, *HIV Medicine,* 9, 452–502.

Dex S. & Joshi H (2005) *Children of the 21st Century: From Birth to Nine Months.* Bristol: Policy Press.

DCSF (2008) *Information sharing: guidance for practitioners and managers,* London: Department for Children, Schools and Families, and Communities and Local Government.

DCSF & Department of Health (2009) *Getting maternity services right for pregnant teenagers and young fathers,* Nottingham, Department for Children Schools and Families.

DCSF, Department of Health, NTA (2009) *Joint Guidance on Development of Local Protocols between Drug and Alcohol Treatment Services and Local Safeguarding and Family Services,* London: Department for Children, Schools and Families (DCSF), Department of Health (DH) and National Treatment Agency for Substance Misuse (NTA)

DfES (2006) *The common assessment framework for children & young people: practitioners' guide,* London, Department for Education and Skills.

DfES (2007) *Every Parent Matters.* Nottingham, Department for Education and Skills.

Doberczak TM, *et al* (1991) Neonatal opiate abstinence syndrome in term and preterm infants, *Journal of Paediatrics,* 118, 6, 933–37.

Doggett C, *et al* (2010) Home visits during pregnancy and after birth for women with an alcohol or drug problem, *Cochrane Database of Systematic Reviews,* Issue 7, The Cochrane Library.

Dolovich LR, *et al* (1998) Benzodiazepine use in pregnancy and major malformations or oral cleft: meta-analysis of cohort and case-control studies. *British Medical Journal,* 317, 839–843.

Draper ES, *et al* (2007) Recreational drug use: a major risk factor for gastroschisis?

American Journal of Epidemiology, December 5 on-line publication.

Dryden C, *et al* (2009) Maternal methadone use in pregnancy: factors associated with the development of neonatal abstinence syndrome and implications for healthcare resources. *British Journal of Obstetrics and Gynaecology*, 116, 665–671.

DrugScope (2010) *Drugsearch index*, London, DrugScope www.drugscope.org.uk accessed on 1 August 2010.

Dysart K, *et al* (2007) Sequela of preterm versus term infants born to mothers on a methadone maintenance program: differential course of neonatal abstinence syndrome, *Journal of Perinatal Medicine*, 35, 344–346.

Effective Interventions Unit, (2002) *Integrated Care for Drug Users*, Edinburgh, Scottish Executive.

Ehrmin JT (2001) Unresolved feelings of guilt and shame in the maternal role with substance-dependent African American women. *Journal of Nursing Scholarship*, 33, 1, 47–52.

Elliott EJ, *et al* (2006) Diagnosis of fetal alcohol syndrome and alcohol use in pregnancy: a survey of paediatrician's knowledge, attitudes and practice, *Journal of Paediatrics and Child Health*, 42, 698–703.

English DR, *et al* (1997) Maternal cannabis use and birth weight: a meta-analysis, *Addiction*, 92, 11, 1553–1560.

Fatherhood Institute (2011) www.fatherhoodinstitute.org

Fergusson DM. *et al* (2002) Maternal use of cannabis and pregnancy outcomes, *British Journal of Obstetrics and Gynaecology*, 109, 21–27.

Forrester D. & Harwin J. (2006) Parental substance misuse and child care social work: findings from the first stage of a study of 100 families, *Child and Family Social Work*, 11, 325–335.

Forrester D. (2007) Patterns of re-referral to social services: a study of 400 closed cases, *Child and Family Social Work*, 12, 11–21.

Frank D, *et al* (1993) Maternal cocaine use: impact on child health and development, *Advances in Pediatrics*, 40, 65–99.

Frank D, *et al* (2001) Growth, Development and behaviour in early childhood following prenatal cocaine exposure: a systematic review. *JAMA*, 285, 12, 1613–1625.

Frank D, *et al* (2002) Forgotten fathers: an exploratory study of mothers' report of drug and alcohol problems among fathers of urban newborns. *Neurotoxicology and Teratology*, 24, 339–347.

French E, et al. (1998) Improving interactions between substance-abusing mothers and their substance-exposed newborns. *Journal of Obstetric Gynecologic & Neonatal Nursing*, 27, 262–269.

Friend KB, *et al* (2004) Alcohol use and sudden infant death syndrome, *Developmental Review*, 24, 235–251.

Fischer B, *et al* (2008) Hepatitis C virus transmission among oral crack users: viral detection on crack paraphernalia, *European Journal of Gastroenterology & Hepatology*, 20,1,29–32.

Fischer G, *et al* (2006) Methadone versus buprenorphine in pregnant addicts: a double-blind, double dummy comparison study, *Addiction*, 101, 275–281.

Geraghty B, et al. (1997) Methadone levels in breast milk. *Journal of Human Lactation*, 13, 3, 227–230.

Gill AC. *et al* (2004) Strabismus in infants of opiate-dependent mothers. *Acta Paediatrics*, 92, 379–385.

Gray R. and Henderson J. (2006) *Review of the fetal effects of prenatal alcohol exposure. Report to the Department of Health*. University of Oxford. National Perinatal Epidemiology Unit.

Gunzerath L. *et al* (2004) National Institute on Alcohol Abuse and Alcoholism report on moderate drinking. *Alcoholism: Clinical and Experimental Research*, 28, 6, 829–847.

Hale TW. (2008) *Medications and mothers' milk: 13th Edition*, Amarillo Texas, Hale Publishing.

Henderson J, *et al* (2007a) Systematic review of effects of low-moderate prenatal alcohol exposure on pregnancy outcome. *British Journal of Obstetrics and Gynaecology*, 114; 243–252.

Henderson J, *et al* (2007b) Systematic review of the fetal effects of prenatal binge-drinking, Journal Epidemiology Community Health, 61, 1069–1073.

Hepburn M. (2004a) Caring for the pregnant drug user, in Beaumont B. (Ed) *Care of Drug Users in General Practice: A harm-minimization approach*, 2nd ed. Oxford, Radcliffe.

Hepburn M. (2004b) Substance abuse in pregnancy, *Current Obstetrics & Gynaecology*, 14, 419–425.

HM Government (2007) *Safe, Sensible, Social: the next steps in the National Alcohol Strategy*, London, Home Office.

HM Government (2008) *Drugs: protecting families and communities. The 2008 Drug Strategy*, London, Home Office.

HM Government (2010a) *Maternity and Early Years – making a good start to family life*, London, Home Office.

HM Government (2010b) *Every Child Matters: change for children*, London, Home Office.

HM Government (2010c) *Working together to safeguard children: a guide to inter-agency working to safeguard and promote the welfare of children*. Nottingham, Department for Children, Schools and Families.

HM Government (2010d) *Drug strategy 2010 – reducing demand, restricting supply, building recovery*, London, Home Office.

Ho E, *et al* (2001) Characteristics of pregnant women who use ecstasy (3,4-methylenedioxymethamphetamine), *Neurotoxicology and Teratology*, 23, 561–567.

Hoddinott P, et al. (2008) Breastfeeding: Clinical Review, *British Medical Journal*, 336, 881–887.

Hogan D. M. (1998) Annotation: the psychological development and welfare of children of opiate and cocaine users: review and research needs. *Journal of Child Psychology and Psychiatry*, 39, 609–620.

Horsley T, *et al* (2007) Benefits and harms associated with the practice of bed sharing: a systematic review, *Archives of Pediatric and Adolescent Medicine*, 161, 237–245.

Hulse GK, *et al* (1997) The relationship between maternal use of heroin and methadone and infant birth weight, *Addiction*, 92, 1571–1579.

Isbister GK, *et al* (2001) Neonatal paroxetine withdrawal syndrome or actually serotonin syndrome? *Archives of Disease in Childhood, Fetal and Neonatal Edition*, 85, F147–148.

Jansson LM, *et al* (2004) Methadone maintenance and lactation: a review of the literature and current management guidelines, *Journal of Human Lactation*, 20, 1, 62–71.

Jansson LM, et al. (2008a) Methadone maintenance and breastfeeding in the neonatal period. *Pediatrics*, 121, 1, 106–114.

Jansson LM, et al. (2008b) Methadone maintenance and long-term lactation, *Breastfeeding Medicine*. 3, 1, 34–37.

Johnson K, *et al* (2003a) Substance misuse during pregnancy. *British Journal of Psychiatry*, 183, 187–189.

Johnson RE, *et al* (2003b) Use of buprenorphine in pregnancy: patient management and effects on the neonate, *Drug and Alcohol Dependence*, 70, 87–101.

Johnstone FD. (1998) Pregnant drug users. IN Robertson JR. (Ed.) *Management of drug users in the community: a practical handbook.* London, Arnold.

Jones HE, et al. (2010) Neonatal Abstinence Syndrome after Methadone or Buprenorphine Exposure, *New England Journal of Medicine*, 363, 2320–2331.

Kakko J, *et al* (2008) Buprenorphine and methadone treatment of opiate dependence during pregnancy: comparison of fetal growth and neonatal outcomes in two consecutive case series. *Drug and Alcohol Dependence*, 96, 69–78.

Kaltenbach KA. (1994) Effects of in-utero opiate exposure: new paradigms for old questions, *Drug and Alcohol Dependence*, 36, 83–87.

Kaner EF. *et al* (2007) Effectiveness of brief interventions in primary care populations. *Cochrane Database of Systematic Reviews*, Issue 2.

Kandall SR, et al. (1993) Relationship of maternal substance abuse to subsequent sudden infant death syndrome in offspring. *Journal of Pediatrics*, 123, 1, 120–126.

Kandall SR, *et al* (1999) The methadone maintained pregnancy, *Clinics in Perinatology*, 26, 1, 173–183.

Klee H. (1998) Drug-using parents: analysing the stereotypes. *International Journal of Drug Policy*, 9, 437–448.

Klee H., *et al* (2002) *Drug misuse and motherhood*, London, Routledge.

Koren G, *et al* (1989) Bias against the null hypothesis: the reproductive hazards of cocaine, *Lancet*, 2, 8677, 1440–1442.

Kraft W, *et al* (2008) Sublingual buprenorphine for treatment of Neonatal Abstinence Syndrome: a randomized trial, *Pediatrics*, 122, e601-e607.

Kroll B. & Taylor A. (2003) *Parental substance misuse and child welfare*, London, Jessica Kingsley.

Kruschel C. (2007) Managing drug withdrawal in the newborn infant, *Seminars in Fetal & Neonatal Medicine*, 12, 127–133.

LaGasse LL, Seifer R, Lester BM. (1999) Interpreting research on prenatal substance exposure in the context of multiple confounding factors. *Clinics in Perinatology*, 26, 39–54.

Lee KG. (2007) Lactation and drugs, *Paediatrics and Child Health*, 17, 2, 68–71.

Lejeune C, *et al* (2006) Prospective multicenter observational study of 260 infants born to 259 opiate-dependent mothers on methadone or high-dose buprenophine substitution, *Drug and Alcohol Dependence*, 82, 250–257.

Lester BM, *et al* (2004) Substance use during pregnancy: time for policy to catch up with research, *Harm Reduction Journal*, 1, 5.

Lewis C. & Lamb M. E. (2007) *Understanding fatherhood: a review of recent research*, York, Joseph Rowntree Foundation.

Lloyd DJ, & Myserscough EJ. (2006) Neonatal Abstinence Syndrome. A new intervention: a community based, structured Health Visitor Assessment. *Substance Misuse Research Programme Report*. Edinburgh, Scottish Executive.

Luty J. *et al* (2003) Is opiate detoxification unsafe in pregnancy? *Journal of Substance Abuse Treatment*, 24, 363–367.

Macrory F. & Crosby S. (1995) Special Care or Segregation?: The need for improvement in the provision of maternity services for drug-using women, paper presented at the *6th International Conference on the Reduction of Drug Related Harm*, Florence, Italy.

Makarechian N, et al. (1998) Association between moderate alcohol consumption during pregnancy and spontaneous abortion, stillbirth and premature birth: A meta-analysis. *Canadian Journal of Clinical Pharmacology*, 5, 3, 169–176.

Malpas TJ, *et al* (1997) Breastfeeding reduces the severity of neonatal abstinence syndrome, *Journal of Paediatrics and Child Health*, 33, 38.

Malpas TJ, & Darlow BA. (1999) Neonatal abstinence syndrome following abrupt cessation of breastfeeding. *New Zealand Medical Journal*, 112, 12 –13.

Martinez FD, *et al* (1994) The effect of paternal smoking on the birth weight of newborns whose mothers did not smoke. *American Journal of Public Health*, 84, 9, 1489–1491.

McCarthy JJ, & Posey BL. (2000) Methadone levels in human milk, *Journal of Human Lactation*, 16, 2, 115–120.

McCarthy JJ. *et al* (2005) High dose methadone maintenance in pregnancy: maternal and neonatal outcomes. *American Journal of Obstetrics and Gynecology*, 193, 3, 606–610.

McElhatton PR. (1994) The effects of benzodiazepine use during pregnancy and lactation, *Reproductive Toxicology*, 8, 6, 461–475.

McKenna JJ, & McDade T. (2005) Why babies should never sleep alone: A review of the co-sleeping controversy in relation to SIDS, bed sharing and breastfeeding, *Paediatric Respiratory Reviews*, 6, 134–152.

McGlothlin WH, *et al* (1970) Effect of LSD on human pregnancy. *JAMA*, 212, 1483–1487.

McMahon T J, *et al* (2008) Drug abuse and responsible fathering: a comparative study of men enrolled in methadone maintenance treatment. *Addiction*, 103, 269–283.

McMahon TJ & Giannini FD (2003) Substance-abusing fathers in family court: moving from popular stereotypes to therapeutic jurisprudence, *Family Court Review*, 41, 3, 337–353.

McMahon TJ, & Rounsaville BJ. (2002) Substance abuse and fathering: adding poppa to the research agenda. *Addiction*, 97, 9, 1109–1115.

Mennella JA & Beauchamp GK. (1991) The transfer of alcohol to human milk: Effects on flavour and the infant's behaviour, *New England Journal of Medicine*, 325, 14, 981–985.

Mennella JA & Gerrish CJ. (1998) Effects of exposure to alcohol in mother's milk on infant sleep, *Pediatrics*, 101, 5, 2.

Messinger DS, *et al* (2004) The Maternal Lifestyle Study: cognitive, motor and behavioural outcomes of cocaine-exposed and opiate-exposed infants through three years of age. *Pediatrics*, 113, 6, 1677–1685.

Meyers RJ, *et al* (2005) The Community Reinforcement Approach: History and Empirical Validation, *Journal of Cognitive Psychotherapy*, 19, 3.

Moran P, *et al* (2009) Substance misuse during pregnancy: its effects and treatment, *Fetal and Maternal Medicine Review*, 20, 1, 1–16.

NHS Health Scotland (2009a) *Ready Steady Baby*, web book accessible on www.readysteadybaby.org.uk

NHS Health Scotland (2009b) *Alcohol Brief Interventions (ABI) Antenatal Pack*, accessible online www.healthscotland.com/documents/4096.aspx

NHS Health Scotland (2009c) *Off to a good start: all you need to know about breastfeeding your baby*, accessible on www.readysteadybaby.org.uk

NHS Information Centre (2007) *Infant Feeding Survey 2005*, The Information Centre for Health and Social Care, www.ic.nhs.uk

NHS Information Centre (2010) *Statistics on Alcohol: England 2010*, The Information Centre for Health and Social Care, www.ic.nhs.uk

NHSQIS (2005) *Clinical Standards – March 2005. Maternity Services*. Edinburgh: NHS Quality Improvement Scotland.

NICE (2006) *Routine postnatal care for women and their babies*, London, National Institute for Health and Clinical Excellence.

NICE (2007a) *Antenatal and postnatal mental health: clinical management and service guidance*, London, National Institute for Health and Clinical Excellence.

NICE (2007b) *Intrapartum care: care of healthy women and their babies during childbirth*, London, National Institute for Health and Clinical Excellence.

NICE (2007c) *Drug misuse: psychosocial interventions. NICE clinical guideline 51.* London, National Institute for Clinical Excellence.

NICE (2007d) *Methadone and buprenorphine for the management of opioid dependence. NICE technology appraisal guidance 114.* London, National Institute for Clinical Excellence.

NICE (2007) *Drug misuse: opioid detoxification. NICE clinical guideline 52.* London, National Institute for Clinical Excellence.

NICE (2008a) *Antenatal care: routine care for the healthy pregnant woman*, London, National Institute for Health and Clinical Excellence.

NICE (2008b) *Improving the nutrition of pregnant and breastfeeding mothers and children in low income households*, London, National Institute for Health and Clinical Excellence.

NICE (2009) *When to suspect child maltreatment: Clinical Guideline*, London, RCOG National Collaborating Centre for Women's and Children's Health.

NICE (2010a) *Care of pregnant women with complex social factors: a model for service provision*, London, National Institute for Health and Clinical Excellence.

NICE (2010b) *How to stop smoking in pregnancy and following childbirth*, London, National Institute for Health and Clinical Excellence.

NTA (2004) *Methadone dose and methadone maintenance treatment. Research into practice 3.* London, National Treatment Agency for Substance Misuse.

NTA (2010) *Women in drug treatment: what the latest figures reveal*, London, National Treatment Agency for Substance Misuse.

NSW Department of Health (2006) *Background papers to the National clinical guidelines for the management of drug use during pregnancy, birth and the early development years of the newborn.* NSW Department of Health, Sydney.

Oei J. and Lui K. (2007) Management of the newborn infant affected by maternal opiates and other drugs of dependency, *Journal of Paediatrics and Child Health*, 43, 9–18.

O'Hare PA, Newcombe R, Matthews A, Buning E.C, & Drucker E. eds (1992) *The reduction of drug-related harm.* Routledge, London.

O'Connor T. (2002) Annotation: The 'effects' of parenting reconsidered: findings, challenges and applications, *Journal of Child Psychology and Psychiatry*, 43, 5, 555–572.

Ornoy A, *et al* (1996) The developmental outcome of children born to heroin-dependent mothers, raised at home or adopted. *Child Abuse and Neglect*, 20, 385–396.

Osborn D, *et al* (2005a) Opiate treatment for opiate withdrawal in newborn infants. *Cochrane Database of Systematic Reviews*, Issue 3.

Osborn D, *et al* (2005b) Sedatives for opiate withdrawal in newborn infants. *Cochrane Database of Systematic Reviews*, Issue 3.

Plant M (1997) *Women and Alcohol: A contemporary and historical perspective*, Free Association Books, London.

Pocock N. (2008) Breastfeeding appears safe for women maintained on methadone, *Pediatrics*, 121, 106–114.

Polygenis D, *et al* (1998) Moderate alcohol consumption during pregnancy and the incidence of fetal malformations: a meta-analysis. *Neurotoxicology and Teratology* 21, 61–67.

Raistrick D, *et al* (2006) *Review of the Effectiveness of Treatment for Alcohol Problems.* National Treatment Agency for Substance Misuse, London.

Robertson JR. Ed (1998) *Management of Drug Users in the Community: A Practical Handbook*, Arnold, London.

Ross A, *et al* (1995) Maternal HIV infection, Drug Use, and Growth of uninfected children in their first 3 years, *Archives of Disease in Childhood*, 73, 6, 490–495.

RCM (2008a) *Woman centred care: Position Statement,* London, Royal College of Midwives.

RCM (2008b) *Hepatitis C Position Statement,* London, Royal College of Midwives.

RCM (2009) *Domestic Abuse in Pregnancy: Position Paper,* London, Royal College of Midwives.

RCM (2010) *Alcohol and pregnancy: Guidance Paper,* London, Royal College of Midwives.

RCOG (2006) *Alcohol consumption and the outcomes of pregnancy. RCOG Statement NO.5.* London, Royal College of Obstetricians & Gynaecologists.

RCOG, RCM, RCA, RCPCH (2008) *Standards for maternity care: report of a working party,* London, Royal College of Obstetricians & Gynaecologists; Royal College of Midwives; Royal College of Anaesthetists; Royal College of Paediatrics and Child Health.

RCOG (2010) *Green-top Guideline NO.39 – Management of HIV in pregnancy,* London, Royal College of Obstetricians & Gynaecologists

Russell M, *et al* (1996) Detecting risk drinking during pregnancy: A comparison of four screening questionnaires. *American Journal of Public Health,* 86, 10, 1435–1439.

Salisbury D, *et al* Eds (2006) *Immunisation against infectious disease: 'The Green Book',* London, Department of Health. www.dh.gov.uk.

SACDM (2008) *Essential Care: A report on the approach required to maximise opportunity for recovery from problem substance use in Scotland,* Edinburgh, Scottish Advisory Committee on Drug Misuse.

Saiki T, *et al* (2010) Neonatal Abstinence Syndrome: postnatal ward versus neonatal unit management, *European Journal of Pediatrics,* 169, 1, 95–98.

Sanz EJ, *et al* (2005) Selective serotonin reuptake inhibitors in pregnant women and neonatal withdrawal syndrome: a database analysis. *Lancet,* 365, 482–487.

Sayal K, *et al* (2009) Binge pattern of alcohol consumption during pregnancy and childhood mental health outcomes: Longitudinal population-based study. *Pediatrics,* 123, e289-e296.

Schempf AH. (2007) Illicit drug use and neonatal outcomes: a critical review, *Obstetrical and Gynecological Survey*, 62, 11, 749–757.

Schempf AH. & Strobino DM. (2008) Illicit Drug Use and Adverse Birth Outcomes: Is It Drugs or Context?, *Journal of Urban Health: Bulletin of the New York Academy of Medicine*, 85, 6, 858–873.

SCIE (2009) Think child, think parent, think family: a guide to parental mental health and child welfare, London, Social Care Institute for Excellence.

Scottish Executive (2001) *A Framework for Maternity Services in Scotland*, Scottish Executive, Edinburgh.

Scottish Executive (2003a) *Getting Our Priorities Right: Good Practice Guidance for working with Children and Families affected by Substance Misuse*, Edinburgh, Scottish Executive.

Scottish Executive (2003b) *Responding to Domestic Abuse: Guidelines for Health Care Workers in NHS Scotland*. Edinburgh.

Scottish Executive (2005) *Getting it right for every child*, Edinburgh, Scottish Executive.

Scottish Government (2008a) *The Road to Recovery: a new approach to tackling Scotland's drug problem*, Edinburgh, Scottish Government.

Scottish Government (2008b) *Early Years Strategy*. Edinburgh, Scottish Government.

Scottish Government (2008c) *Equally Well: Report of the Scottish Government Ministerial Task Force on Health Inequalities*, Edinburgh, Scottish Government.

Scottish Government (2009a) *Changing Scotland's relationship with alcohol: A framework for action*, Edinburgh, Scottish Government.

Scottish Government (2009b) *Enhanced maternity services for women within NHS Scotland*, Edinburgh, Scottish Government.

Scottish Government (2010a) *Guidelines for services providing injecting equipment*. Edinburgh, Scottish Government.

Scottish Government (2010b) *National guidance for child protection in Scotland*, Edinburgh, Scottish Government.

Scottish Government (2011) *Improving maternal and infant nutrition: A framework for action*, Edinburgh, Scottish Government.

Seligman NS, *et al* (2010) Relationship between maternal methadone dose at delivery and neonatal abstinence syndrome, *Journal of Pediatrics*, 157, 428–433.

Shaw NJ. & McIvor L. (1994) Neonatal abstinence syndrome after maternal methadone treatment, *Archives Diseases Childhood*, 71, F203-F205.

Shaw A, *et al* (2007) Drugs and poverty: a literature review. *A report for the Scottish Association of Alcohol and Drug Action Teams*. Glasgow, Scottish Drugs Forum (SDF).

Shenassa ED. & Brown MJ. (2004) Maternal smoking and infantile gastrointestinal dysregulation: the case of colic. *Pediatrics*, 114, 4, 497–505.

Sidebotham P. (2001) An ecological approach to child abuse: a creative use of scientific models in research and practice. *Child Abuse Review*, 10, 97–112.

SIGN (2002) *Postnatal Depression and Puerperal Psychosis*, Scottish Intercollegiate Guidelines Network. www.sign.ac.uk

SIGN (2003) *The Management of Harmful Drinking and Alcohol Dependence in Primary Care: A National Clinical Guideline*, Scottish Intercollegiate Guidelines Network. www.sign.ac.uk

SIGN (2006) *Management of hepatitis C: A national clinical guideline NO.92*. Scottish Intercollegiate Guidelines Network. www.sign.ac.uk

Siney C. Ed (1999) *Pregnancy and Drug Misuse*, Books for Midwives Press, Cheshire.

Smith EJ. *et al* (2009) Pharmacologic interventions for pregnant women enrolled in alcohol treatment. *Cochrane Database of Systematic Reviews*, Issue 3.

Smith LM, *et al* (2008) Prenatal methamphetamine use and neonatal neurobehavioural outcome, *Neurotoxicology and Teratology*, 30, 20–28.

Sokol RJ, *et al* (1989) The T-ACE questions: Practical prenatal detection of risk drinking. *American Journal of Obstetrics and Gynecology*,160, 4, 863–870.

Street K, *et al* (2008) Is adequate parenting compatible with maternal drug use? A five year follow-up. *Child care health and development*, 34, 2, 204–206.

Templeton L, *et al* (2006) *Looking Beyond Risk: Parental substance misuse scoping study. Final report to the Scottish Executive.* Edinburgh, Substance Misuse Research programme, Scottish Executive.

Terplan M. & Lui S. (2007) Psychosocial interventions for pregnant women in outpatient illicit drug treatment programs compared to other interventions. *Cochrane Database of Systematic Reviews*, Issue 4.

Topley J. *et al* (2007) Behavioural, developmental and child protection outcomes following exposure to class A drugs in pregnancy, *Child: care, health and development*, 34, 1, 71–76.

Tran TT (2009) Management of hepatitis B in pregnancy: weighing the options, *Cleveland Clinic Journal of Medicine*, 76, 3, S25-S29.

Tunnard J (2002a) Parental drug misuse – a review of impact and intervention studies. *research in practice*. Darlington. www.rip.org.uk

Tunnard J (2002b) Parental problem drinking and its impact on children, *research in practice*, Darlington. www.rip.org.uk

Tunnard J (2004) Parental mental health problems: key messages from research, policy and practice, *research in practice*, Darlington. www.rip.org.uk

Underdown A, *et al* (2009) Massage intervention for promoting mental and physical health in infants aged under six months, *Cochrane Database of Systematic Reviews*, The Cochrane Library, Issue 4.

U.S. Department of Health and Human Services (2000) *National Institute on Alcohol Abuse and Alcoholism. Tenth special report to the U.S. Congress on alcohol and health: Highlights from current research.* Washington, DC: The Institute.

U.S. Department of Health and Human Services (2006) *The Health Consequences of Involuntary Exposure to Tobacco Smoke: A Report of the Surgeon General*, Atlanta, U.S. Department of Health and Human Services, Centers for Disease Control and Prevention, Coordinating Center for Health Promotion, National Center for Chronic Disease Prevention and Health Promotion, Office on Smoking and Health.

Velleman R. & Templeton L. (2007) Understanding and modifying the impact of parents' substance misuse on children. *Advances in Psychiatric Treatment*, 13, 79–89.

Ward J, *et al* (1998) *Methadone Maintenance Therapy and Other Opioid Replacement Therapies*, Harwood Academic Publishers, New Jersey.

Welsh Assembly Government (2008) *Working together to reduce harm: the substance misuse strategy for Wales 2008–2018*, Cardiff, Welsh Assembly Government.

Whittaker A & McLeod J (1998) in Robertson JR, (Ed) *Management of Drug Users in the Community: A Practical Handbook*, Arnold, London.

Wilbourne PL, *et al* (2000) Benzodiazepine and methadone use is associated with longer neonatal withdrawal in poly-substance exposed infants. *American Journal of Obstetrics & Gynecology*, 182, 1, 2, S177.

Winklbaur B, *et al* (2008) Treating pregnant women dependent on opioids is not the same as treating pregnancy and opioid dependence: a knowledge synthesis for better treatment for women and neonates, *Addiction*, 103, 1429–1440.

Wojnar-Horton RE, et al. (1997) Methadone distribution and excretion into breast milk of clients in a methadone maintenance programme, *British Journal of Pharmacology*, 44, 543–547.

WHO (1992) *International Statistical Classification of Diseases and related health problems. 10th Edition.* Geneva, World Health Organization.

WHO (1996) *Hepatitis B and breastfeeding: Update No. 22*, Geneva, World Health Organization.

WHO (1997) *Cannabis: a health perspective and research agenda*, Geneva, World Health Organization.

WHO (2003) *Global strategy for infant and young child feeding*, Geneva, World Health Organization.

WHO (2006) *Child maltreatment and alcohol*, Geneva, World Health Organization.

WHO (2008) *HIV transmission through breastfeeding: A review of available evidence 2007 update*, Geneva, World Health Organization.

WHO, UNODC & UNAIDS (2004) *Position Paper: Substitution maintenance therapy in the management of opioid dependence and HIV/AIDS prevention*, Geneva, World Health Organization, United Nations Office on Drugs and Crime, Joint United Nations Programme on HIV/AIDS.

Wikner BN, *et al* (2007) Use of benzodiazepines and benzodiazepine receptor agonists during pregnancy: neonatal outcome and congenital malformations, *Pharmacoepidemiology Drug Safety*, 16, 1203–1210.

Witkiewitz K, & Marlatt GA. (2004) Relapse Prevention for Alcohol and Drug Problems. *American Psychologist*, 59, 4, 224–235.

Wittman B, & Segal S. (1991) A comparison of the effects of single and split dose methadone administration on the foetus: ultrasound examination. *International Journal of Addiction*, 26, 213–218.

Wright A & Walker J (2007) Management of women who use drugs during pregnancy, *Seminars in Fetal and Neonatal Medicine*, 12, 114–118.

Appendix 1

To access this leaflet as a printable document, please go to www.drugscope.org.uk/pregnancyguide

Model care pathway

	Pre-conception care ↓	• Advice on reproductive health, fertility, contraception, sexual health and family planning • Review tobacco, alcohol, and drug use • Advice on pregnancy care, nutrition, folic acid, Vitamin D • Review BBV risk and offer testing
	Confirmation of pregnancy / first contact with health professional ↓	• Arrange booking appointment with community midwifery team (self-referral or professional referral) • Woman to attend GP (e.g. healthy lifestyle advice, folic acid, food hygiene) • Arrange scan for 12 weeks
10 weeks	BOOKING appointment Multi-disciplinary information sharing /initial child care risk assessment ↓	• Follow antenatal care pathway • Complete maternity liaison form (problem substance use) • Smoking cessation advice and support • Alcohol brief interventions if required • Refer to drug/alcohol specialist if required • Refer to specialist midwifery service for problem substance use / book appointment with obstetrician • Give leaflet 'Pregnant... and using alcohol or drugs?' • Give leaflet 'Caring for a baby with drug withdrawal symptoms' • BBV testing (HIV & HBV, HCV if at-risk). • If positive, follow agreed BBV care pathway • 'Infant feeding' checklist and advice re breastfeeding • Assess social circumstances, discuss maternity benefits • Risk assessment (child protection issues) • Consent for sharing information and inter-agency working • Give woman handheld maternity records • 'The Pregnancy Book', 'Ready Steady Baby' • If woman does not attend booking – follow-up by midwife
12 weeks	↓	• Scan and 1st trimester screening (if consented)
16 weeks	Antenatal appointment Implement maternity care plan ↓	• Discuss assessment and care needs with obstetrician • Discuss and agree maternity care plan • Discuss and agree management of drug/alcohol use with specialists • Identify lead person to organise multi-agency assessment and family support plan meeting
20 weeks	↓	• Fetal anomaly scan

To access this leaflet as a printable document, please go to www.drugscope.org.uk/pregnancyguide

22 weeks	Antenatal appointment ↓	• Monitor progress including drug/alcohol use • Arrange multi-agency meeting with parents/professionals • Home visit assessment – include safe storage of drugs discussion
24 weeks	Multi-agency meeting and family support plan ↓	• Multi-agency meeting with parents to discuss assessment and agree a 'family support plan' • Review drug/alcohol use and treatment plan • Discuss parenting capacity of mother and father • Discuss care of baby with NAS/FAS • Appoint 'Lead Professional' to co-ordinate family support plan
28 weeks	Antenatal appointment ↓	• Child protection case conference (if required) and child protection care plan (if required) • Growth scan / fetal monitoring if required • Discuss birth plan
32 weeks	Antenatal appointment ↓	• Start preparation for parenthood • Assess fetal growth – 2nd growth scan • Discuss labour and delivery (include protocol re prescription) • Discuss and agree postnatal contraception • Monitor drug/alcohol use – update maternity liaison form
36 weeks	Antenatal appointment ↓	• Preparation for parenthood • Assess fetal growth • Discuss care of baby with NAS/FAS
38 weeks	Antenatal appointment	• Preparation for parenthood • Monitor drug/alcohol use
Term (40 weeks)	CHILDBIRTH ↓	• If undelivered, see woman at 40 weeks and 41 weeks and plan induction of labour • If delivered, follow postnatal care pathway • Breastfeeding support and advice • Postnatal contraception • Parenting support for mother and father • Neonatal Abstinence Syndrome (NAS) assessment and care if required • Fetal Alcohol Syndrome (FAS) assessment and care if required • Discharge planning multi-agency meeting (include prescription arrangements in care plan) • Review and update Family Support Plan • Identify lead professional/care co-ordinator for postnatal care plan • Discharge pack – discuss reducing the risk of SIDS (cot death) and bed-sharing

To access this leaflet as a printable document, please go to www.drugscope.org.uk/pregnancyguide

| 10 days | Postnatal care

Review family support plan/ child protection plan as required

↓ | • Continue inter-agency support / postnatal care plan
• Continue NAS / FAS assessment and care (if required)
• Reassess drug / alcohol use following discharge
• Relapse prevention support
• Parenting support for mother and father
• Midwife ends care (day 10 to 28)
• Complete maternity liaison form (problem substance use) to document pregnancy outcomes
• Home visit by health visitor day 11 onwards
• Arrange multi-agency review meeting date in 6-8 weeks time |

Appendix 2

To access this leaflet as a printable document, please go to www.drugscope.org.uk/pregnancyguide

Keeping children safe from alcohol and drugs in the home

It is important to make sure that infants, children and young people are kept safe from alcohol and drugs that adults use and keep in the home. A number of children in the UK have died or nearly died as a result of adults exposing children to dangerous drugs. Over half of all poisoning cases in children are caused by them swallowing medication/drugs.

Please read this leaflet and discuss it with your healthcare professional.

Keep children safe

Children are naturally curious and do not understand danger. Alcohol and drugs may look very attractive to a young child. Don't expect them to know the difference between brightly coloured drugs or alcoholic drinks and sweets or fizzy drinks.

Methadone and other drugs

Even a very tiny amount of methadone can kill a child. If a child swallows methadone, they can stop breathing and they can choke on their own saliva or vomit because they cannot swallow when they are very drowsy or unconscious.

Please take these simple steps to store your methadone, and any other drugs that you have in the home, SAFELY:

- Put your drugs away as soon as you bring them home and every time after you use/take them. Always keep them out of sight and out of reach. Keep them in a high cupboard that can be locked or high up in a locked wardrobe.
- If you don't have a lockable cupboard or wardrobe, please buy a padlock or a lockable and unbreakable container like a cashbox.
- If you don't have somewhere to lock away your drugs, then make sure they are kept somewhere high up, where they cannot be seen or reached by climbing.

Prescribed medication like methadone and diazepam

Make sure your pharmacist puts your medication – whether tablets, capsules or liquid – into a bottle with a child-resistant cap. These caps can save lives, *but*

To access this leaflet as a printable document, please go to www.drugscope.org.uk/pregnancyguide

remember, they are not 100% child-proof, they can be opened – even by small children. Keep them out of sight and out of reach.

Never store your drugs in a different container from the one you are given by the pharmacist. Always return any left over medicines to your pharmacist. Never keep them in the house.

Never – not even for a minute – leave drugs:

✗   On the floor
✗   In a bag, handbag or coat pocket
✗   Under a bed
✗   In a child's bedroom
✗   In the bathroom
✗   Down the back of a sofa
✗   On top of a table
✗   In a car glove-box
✗   In the fridge
✗   Unattended when travelling with children

Taking medicine and other drugs in the home

✔   When you take your methadone or any other medicine, make sure you take exactly the right dose.
✔   Avoid taking drugs in front of children.
✔   Put drugs away straight after use. Don't leave them on a table or work surface.
✔   If you accidentally spill your methadone (or any other drug), clear it up immediately. Wash any cloth or safely dispose of any paper towel you use for cleaning up. Just putting them in the bin may mean children are at risk as they could easily get them out again!
✔   When you finish your bottle of methadone or other medicine, remember to rinse out the bottle with water before disposing of it.

If you buy methadone or other drugs *off the street* remember:

●   You cannot be sure of the strength or the purity - or even if it is the drug or medicine that you have been told it is!
●   They may not be in bottles with child-resistant lids.

To access this leaflet as a printable document, please go to www.drugscope.org.uk/pregnancyguide

- If a child swallows them you and the doctor may not be able to tell what they have taken.

Talking to children about the dangers of drugs

If you have children, or look after children, talk to them about the dangers of taking alcohol or drugs or any medicine that's not for them. Keep all your medicines, drugs and alcohol 'out of sight' and 'out of reach' and tell your children never to touch any bottles of alcohol or medicine that are in the home. Tell children that if they ever take any drugs or alcohol by mistake to tell you straight away so you can help them.

What to do if a child takes drugs

If you suspect a child or young person has consumed alcohol or taken a drug by accident, lie them on their side in the **recovery position** (see picture below), **dial 999 straight away**, and stay with the child until the ambulance arrives to take them to the nearest accident and emergency unit. If possible, get someone else to call 999 while you stay with the child.

Tell the medical professional what the child has taken, how much, when, and how quickly (show them the bottle if possible). Do not try and make the child sick, and do not try and make the child drink if they are drowsy.

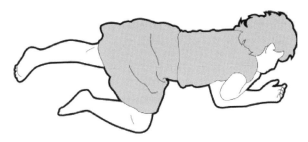

To put someone in the recovery position, follow these steps:
1. Place the arm nearest to you at right angles to the body, elbow bent.
2. Bring the far arm across the chest, and hold the back of the person's hand against their nearest cheek.

*Diagram reproduced with kind permission of ©The British Red Cross.

To access this leaflet as a printable document, please go to www.drugscope.org.uk/pregnancyguide

3. Grasp the far leg just above the knee and pull it up, keeping the foot on the ground.
4. Keeping the hand pressed against the cheek, pull on the far leg to roll the person towards you onto their side.
5. Adjust the upper leg so that both the hip and the knee are at right angles.
6. Tilt the head back, and lift the chin forward, to make sure the person's airway (mouth and throat) remain open. If necessary, adjust the hand under the cheek to keep the head tilted.
7. Check person cannot roll forwards or backwards.
8. If the person has to stay in the recovery position for more than 30 minutes, turn them on their opposite side.
9. Keep an eye on the person's breathing and pulse.

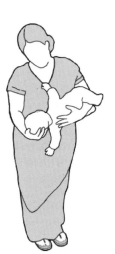

Recovery position for an infant (babies less than 1 year old)

If an infant is unconscious but breathing,
- cradle the infant in your arms,
- place them on their side with their head tilted downwards to prevent them choking on their tongue or inhaling vomit.
- dial 999 and check for vital signs – breathing, pulse and level of response until medical help arrives.

*Diagram reproduced with kind permission of ©The British Red Cross.

Injecting drugs – risks to children

You need to make sure that others are not put at risk by the unsafe use and disposal of injecting equipment.
- Children should never witness you or others injecting drugs.
- Children do not have the same understanding of danger as adults do. They may not be frightened of seeing needles or works, and they may attempt to pick them up or touch them.

- If you or someone else is injecting drugs in the home, keep the sharps bin (cin bin) in a locked secure place out of reach and out of sight of children.
- Make sure all injecting equipment is put away as soon as you get home and disposed of, or put away, immediately after you use it. Keep your equipment in a high cupboard that can be locked or high up in a locked wardrobe.
- Warn children never to touch needles and syringes. If you find them on the street or in your neighbourhood – **do not pick them up**. You can call your Local Council's Environmental Health Department to ask them to pick up needles and syringes left in public places.

Safe disposal of injecting equipment

All used equipment can be disposed of in a sharps bin, this includes: needles, filters, swabs, tissues, spoons, foil, crack pipes, Citric and Vitamin C sachets, water amps etc. The sharps bin can then be returned to your local needle exchange or pharmacy.

Needle-stick injury

It is important to be aware of the risks caused by infections which can be passed on in the blood by injecting or by a needle-stick injury. **HIV, hepatitis C, hepatitis B** and other infections can be passed on this way.

Emergency action – needle-stick injury

If you think a child has jabbed themselves with a needle, you should:
- Encourage bleeding by squeezing the site of the injury
- Wash thoroughly with soap and water
- Cover up with a plaster to prevent germs from entering the wound
- Seek medical attention immediately. Don't panic, but it is important that they get checked out as quickly as possible as they may need treatment.

To access this leaflet as a printable document, please go to www.drugscope.org.uk/pregnancyguide

Safety checklist – important things to remember:

- Store drugs safely in the home – locked away, out of sight, out of reach
- Avoid taking drugs in front of children
- Do not put medicines in bottles without child-resistant lids
- Teach children about the dangers of medicines/drugs/alcohol that are not for them
- Never give children drugs like methadone – you will endanger their life
- Take old or unwanted medicines to a pharmacy for safe disposal
- Store and dispose of injecting equipment safely
- Keep this leaflet safe and read from time to time.

Always discuss storing your medication/ drugs/ alcohol safely with your doctor, nurse, pharmacist, health visitor or midwife. They will help you plan how to store substances safely, and will talk to you more about the information in this leaflet so that you can KEEP CHILDREN SAFE.

Appendix 3

To access this leaflet as a printable document, please go to www.drugscope.org.uk/pregnancyguide

Family support plan:
Children affected by parental substance use

Details of MOTHER

Name   Date of birth

Address

Postcode   Telephone

Details of FATHER

Name   Date of birth

Address

Postcode   Telephone

Details of other parents/ carers including kinship carers

Name   Date of birth

Address

Postcode   Telephone

Details of all CHILDREN:

Unborn baby? Yes ☐ No ☐ If yes, estimated date of delivery: / /

Plan written by: Date:

Name of lead professional appointed to co-ordinate the delivery of this family support plan:

Plan co-ordinated by: Date:

Family support plan:
Children affected by parental substance use

Name of all professionals involved with family members	Agency/Service	Contact details	Frequency of contact e.g. weekly for 1 hour

To access this leaflet as a printable document, please go to www.drugscope.org.uk/pregnancyguide

Family support plan: Children affected by parental substance use

Identified needs	Agreed action/intervention to address needs (include what, where, who, when, why and how)	Desired outcome/goal	Timescale

Contingency Plan (What will happen if the plan is not adhered to or expected outcomes are not achieved?)

Date of next review: _____

Appendix 4

To access this leaflet as a printable document, please go to www.drugscope.org.uk/pregnancyguide

Pregnant... and using alcohol or drugs?

Information to help you, your baby and your family

Knowing about the effects of tobacco, alcohol and drug use during pregnancy is important. This booklet provides you with some information and advice to help you and your baby stay as healthy as possible and to help you prepare for the birth of your baby.

Tobacco, alcohol and drug use during pregnancy

You might be feeling worried about how your alcohol or drug use could affect your pregnancy and baby. It is important to remember that most women who use alcohol and drugs have a normal pregnancy and a perfectly healthy baby. However, there are risks associated with tobacco, alcohol and drug use. Reducing these risks could be helpful to both you and your baby.

Unfortunately, good evidence on the effects of alcohol and drug use during pregnancy has been difficult to establish. What we do know however, is that **smoking tobacco** during pregnancy (or being exposed to tobacco smoke) is definitely harmful to your unborn baby and can negatively affect your pregnancy in a number of ways. We advise all pregnant women (and their partners) who smoke cigarettes to try to give up and we provide a lot of help for you to do this! Ask your midwife, GP, or pharmacist for help.

Smoking tobacco, using street drugs (like heroin, cocaine or crack), injecting drugs or being dependent on drugs (like methadone or valium) can all increase your chances of having a preterm (premature) birth and a low birth weight (small) baby. This in turn can lead to other problems. The risk of *cot death* (Sudden Infant Death Syndrome or 'SIDS') is also increased.

There is no good evidence to suggest that illicit (street) drugs, or drugs like methadone, cause birth defects. However, babies born to **women who drink too much alcohol** during pregnancy can be born with birth defects and brain damage. This in turn, can lead to serious long term problems for children. Even low to moderate levels of alcohol have been linked to an increased risk of miscarriage and no 'safe' level of alcohol use during pregnancy has ever really been established. We therefore advise all pregnant women to avoid alcohol during the first 3 months of pregnancy and preferably up until the baby is born. If you do drink alcohol during pregnancy, we recommend drinking no more than 1-2 units of alcohol once or twice a week. Speak to your midwife, GP or health worker to work out how many units are in alcoholic drinks.

Tobacco and heavy **crack/ cocaine** use are linked to a number of problems in pregnancy because these drugs reduce oxygen and blood flow to the unborn baby, and they can affect the placenta in a number of ways. **Injecting drugs** carries a lot more risks for you and your baby, especially the risk of infections and preterm delivery.

Little is known about the harmful effects of other drugs such as cannabis ('hash'), amphetamines ('speed'), ecstasy, solvents ('gas' and 'glue'), LSD ('acid') and other 'designer' drugs or 'legal highs'. However, the advice is that when in doubt about the effect of a drug, it is best to avoid during pregnancy. Street drugs may contain impurities and can put extra strain on your liver and kidneys, so it is better if you can use **only drugs that have been prescribed to you** when you are pregnant.

It is important to remember that there are many things that can affect your pregnancy, not just tobacco, alcohol and drugs. For instance, the food you eat (your diet), your lifestyle and social circumstances, and whether or not you get good antenatal (maternity) care. Alcohol and drug use can affect your appetite, weight, dental health, general health, mood, relationships and ability to cope with everyday life.

Changing your drug use when pregnant

If you are using opiate drugs (e.g. methadone, dihydrocodeine, buprenorphine or heroin) try to keep your drug use as stable as possible throughout your pregnancy. This means taking the same amount of drug every day and avoiding getting 'stoned' or taking extra, as far as you can. Remember: remaining on prescribed drugs like methadone right the way through pregnancy is perfectly OK if that is what helps you to keep stable and well. It is not appropriate for anyone to tell you that you MUST come off methadone when pregnant.

If you are injecting drugs you will be given help to try and stop or cut down. If you are dependent on heroin you will be advised to take prescribed opiates instead (e.g. methadone). Seek help from specialist drug services. They will see you very quickly if you are pregnant.

To access this leaflet as a printable document, please go to www.drugscope.org.uk/pregnancyguide

If you are prescribed drugs like methadone, and experience morning sickness, we normally recommend splitting your daily dose into two or more lots (e.g. one dose in the morning and one at night). Splitting up your dose will keep you and your baby more stable late in pregnancy too.

Reducing... if you think you could manage to reduce your drug use a bit then you will be supported to do so. Talk to your doctor or drug worker first, so you can do this sensibly. It is important to avoid relapse, so slow reductions over a number of weeks or months are normally recommended. If you are taking benzodiazepines (e.g. valium) you will be given help to reduce these first. If you are reducing your intake of drugs it is advisable to see your drug worker every week so that they can keep a close eye on your progress.

Stopping... it is generally safe to stop using cannabis ('hash'), cocaine or 'crack', amphetamines ('speed'), ecstasy, solvents ('gas' and 'glue'), LSD or 'acid' and other 'designer' drugs. We normally suggest stopping all these drugs during pregnancy. If you cannot stop taking stimulant drugs (e.g. cocaine, 'crack' or 'speed') then get help as soon as you can, because heavy use of these drugs during pregnancy tends to lead to a number of complications. Stopping tobacco smoking at any time during pregnancy can be good for the baby so ask for help whenever you feel ready to stop.

Some woman who are dependent on opiates or benzodiazepines consider stopping their drug use altogether. If you think you might want to do this then you should speak with your doctor or specialist drug worker. DO NOT suddenly stop taking opiates (e.g. heroin, methadone, dihydrocodeine or buprenorphine) or benzodiazepines (e.g. valium) as this could be risky for you and your baby. If you want to come off, it is best done under medical supervision, so that your unborn baby can be checked and you can be given support. If you are dependent on both opiates and benzodiazepines, we would normally help you to come off benzodiazepines first, as these drugs can cause more problems for the baby than opiates.

Alcohol... heavy drinking during pregnancy (including 'binge' drinking) can be very harmful to your baby. If you are drinking more than 2 standard drinks (or 3 units) every day and can't stop or reduce your drinking, then talk to your midwife or doctor who can arrange specialist help. If you are drinking heavily (more than 5 standard drinks a day – or 7.5 units) then you should get help straight away. Pregnant women who are alcohol dependent (addicted to alcohol) will be seen very quickly and are normally offered treatment - a 'detox' - to help them stop drinking. Talk to your midwife, GP or a healthcare professional about your alcohol use in more detail.

Effects of alcohol and drugs after the baby is born

If you are dependent on certain drugs the baby will be born dependent on these too, and can develop what is known as 'Neonatal Abstinence Syndrome'. This is a condition where the baby shows signs and symptoms of withdrawal (usually within 3 days of birth). It can happen with alcohol, benzodiazepine drugs (e.g. valium), and opiates (e.g. methadone, dihydrocodeine, buprenorphine or heroin). At birth, the baby's drug supply stops and the baby goes through a period of withdrawal. Baby withdrawals usually last a few days or weeks, but they can go on for a number of months.

It is difficult to predict how each baby will react. It depends on what drugs you have been taking, how much and for how long. It also depends on the way your body deals with the drugs you are taking (your metabolism during pregnancy), the gestational age of the baby (how far the pregnancy has gone when the baby is born), and the baby's ability to clear the drugs from their system.

It is important to remember that there is no clear link between the *amount* of drugs you take and whether or not the baby will be affected after it is born. This means that even if you reduce your intake of drugs before the birth, the baby may develop withdrawal symptoms. In the same way, some babies born to mothers who are on high doses of drugs like methadone do not always develop severe symptoms. This is why we like to prepare all parents just in case.

Antenatal care (before the birth)

When you are pregnant it is very important that you are checked regularly and attend for all your appointments, scans and other tests. Women (and their babies), who get regular antenatal checks tend to do better than those who don't, regardless of what drugs they are taking.

Midwives and obstetricians (maternity doctors) are there to help and will try to answer any questions and fears that you may have. When you see the midwife, talk to them about your tobacco, alcohol and drug use so that you can be offered the special care that you, your baby and your family need.

To access this leaflet as a printable document, please go to www.drugscope.org.uk/pregnancyguide

If you have a drug or alcohol worker, tell them you are pregnant so that they can help you manage your substance use during pregnancy. You might also need support from a social worker or welfare rights worker to help with benefits or any other social issues (e.g. housing, debts, legal problems, employment issues etc). You might also need support from children's services to help with child care, especially if you have other children to look after, or if it is your first baby and you don't have much support from family and friends.

Normally, the midwife will organise a professionals' meeting when you are around 6-7 months pregnant to discuss how things are going and to plan ahead for the arrival of your baby. You and your partner will be invited to attend this meeting. Ideally, this should ensure that all the professionals involved in your care are clear about what support you and your family need, what outcomes or goals you are working towards, and what services can be provided for the family. Normally a 'named person' or 'lead professional' will work with you to ensure everything goes according to plan.

Sometimes there are concerns about a parent's, or both parents, ability to cope with a newborn baby and there are possible risks to the unborn baby's well-being and safety. In these circumstances, Social Services normally take the lead in planning care for the family and may organise a child protection case conference and may set up a child protection care plan **before** the baby is born. Either way, you should be clear about what support is in place for you and the family well before the birth.

HIV, hepatitis B and hepatitis C

Your midwife will offer routine testing for HIV and hepatitis B at your antenatal 'booking' appointment. These infections can pass from mother to baby. Treatment can now greatly reduce the likelihood of your baby getting these infections so it is important you get tested. If you have injected drugs or had unprotected sex (sex without a condom) with anyone who has injected drugs, you could be at risk of HIV, hepatitis B and hepatitis C. Your midwife or GP will normally offer testing for hepatitis C if you have been at risk. We also recommend that you get immunised (vaccinated) for hepatitis B. If you (or your partner) are injecting drugs we recommend that the whole household gets immunised. Unfortunately there is no immunisation available against HIV and hepatitis C.

To access this leaflet as a printable document, please go to www.drugscope.org.uk/pregnancyguide

Labour and childbirth

Most women who use alcohol or drugs have a normal labour and a normal delivery. The obstetrician (maternity doctor) and paediatrician (child doctor) will get involved if there are any complications. Some women worry about whether or not they will be given enough pain relief... you don't need to worry. You will get to take your prescribed drugs as normal in hospital and you will also be given additional pain relief when you need it. It is important that hospital staff know what drugs you are taking (including any street drugs), as this will affect what pain relief is given (for instance there are some pain relief drugs that don't work with methadone, heroin and dihydrocodeine).

You need to let maternity staff know the name, address and telephone number of your pharmacist (chemist) and prescribing doctor. It is hospital policy to cancel prescriptions before giving drugs (such as methadone) in the maternity wards. You should take all your medication into hospital with you and give it to the staff. This way, you will avoid any problems or delays in getting the medication that you need in hospital.

Postnatal care (after the birth)

Mothers with drug or alcohol problems are asked to stay in hospital (in the postnatal ward) for at least 3 days (72 hours) after the baby is born so that the baby's condition can be checked. In the postnatal ward you will be expected to look after your baby at all times. You will have a chance to start bonding with your baby and you will get some childcare and breastfeeding support. Following the birth, the changes in your body can mean that your normal dose of prescribed drug affects you more than usual. This is something to be careful of as over-sedation (feeling 'stoned') may mean that you could accidentally drop your baby or not hear them crying.

Before you and your baby can be discharged from hospital, the staff will want to review the care plan for your family, and if necessary make some changes if needed. This will depend on how well your baby is doing and how well you and your partner are coping. Babies are not discharged home unless everyone is happy that the baby will be well looked after.

To access this leaflet as a printable document, please go to www.drugscope.org.uk/pregnancyguide

After you leave the postnatal ward with your baby, the midwife will visit you at home. When your baby is 11 days old, your health visitor will visit and will be a good source of information and support on parenthood and all aspects of health for you and your baby. There will be baby clinics in your local area where the growth and development of your child will be assessed and you can meet other parents. Most areas also have breastfeeding support groups, baby massage groups and parent and child groups to go to as well. It is important that you know about what services are available for you and your family.

The time after the baby is born can be difficult for some mothers and fathers. Tiredness, lack of sleep, the 'baby blues', and other stresses (like the baby still having some withdrawal symptoms) can make it harder to look after your baby. This is normal and your midwife, health visitor, doctor and drug/alcohol worker are there to offer support.

Breastfeeding

Breastfeeding has lots of benefits for the long-term health and development of your baby. It helps to promote bonding, and it helps to calm babies who develop withdrawal symptoms. You will be given lots of encouragement to breastfeed. The exception to this would be if you were HIV positive because babies can be infected with HIV through breastfeeding.

In most cases, the benefits of breastfeeding outweigh any worries about continued drug use. However, the midwife or obstetrician will discuss the risks involved in breastfeeding if you are injecting, using street drugs, drinking alcohol heavily or taking any other drugs/medication that might pose a problem for breastfeeding. There is no evidence that hepatitis C is passed to the baby through breastfeeding, so even if you are hepatitis C positive you will be encouraged to breastfeed.

If you are prescribed methadone, it is important to know that only a small amount of the drug is passed to the baby through breast milk, even if you are taking high doses. If you do successfully breastfeed and continue to take drugs like methadone you will be advised to slowly wean the baby onto solids when the time is right. Your health visitor can give you advice about this.

If you smoke cigarettes, drink alcohol or take drugs, there is one very important thing to remember about feeding your baby – **NEVER share a bed with your baby - and NEVER feed your baby lying down in bed, on a sofa, on the**

floor, or in a chair where you could fall asleep and suffocate or injure your baby. We advise parents to always let their baby sleep safely on their back in a cot. The midwife and health visitor will talk to you about the risks of bed-sharing and will also discuss cot death and ways to reduce the risk of cot death.

Professional help

A number of healthcare professionals, along with your GP, may be involved in the care of you and your baby. *Midwives* are specially trained in pregnancy and childbirth. *Obstetricians* are doctors who care for women in pregnancy and childbirth. *Neonatologists* are doctors who care for newborn babies. *Paediatricians* are doctors who care for infants, children and young people. *Health visitors* are specially trained in child and family health. All are keen to involve fathers.

Specialist drug and/or alcohol services are able to offer you a lot of help whilst you are pregnant and after your baby is born. Ask your GP or midwife for advice about how to contact them. Specialist services give priority to pregnant woman and will see you very quickly. Drug and alcohol services also understand the importance of helping fathers-to-be who have drug and/or alcohol problems and will want to offer them a similar service. If your partner has problems related to alcohol or drugs then tell them to speak to their own GP or the midwife, who can arrange help.

Getting support

It is very important that you get all the help and support you need during your pregnancy and beyond. Show this leaflet to your partner and any other person (family or friends) who will be supporting you to look after your baby. There are a lot of myths about drug use during pregnancy and a lot of bad feelings towards mothers who use alcohol or drugs so it is important you get sound information and have a positive experience.

Some parents worry that their baby may be 'taken into care' just because they have an alcohol or drug problem. Drug or alcohol use on its own is not a reason to involve the Social Work Department or to assume you cannot care for your baby properly. However, if there are concerns about the welfare or safety of your child, or if the social work department can help the family, then they may need to do an assessment and get involved. This is the same policy for everyone, whether or not they use alcohol or drugs.

To access this leaflet as a printable document, please go to www.drugscope.org.uk/pregnancyguide

In the UK we have a good system of health and social care that works well with people who use drugs or alcohol. Everyone is interested in your wellbeing and the wellbeing of your baby and family, and we want to make your experience of pregnancy and childbirth a happy one.

Please feel free to speak to a healthcare professional about the information in this leaflet, especially if there is anything that you don't understand or would like to talk about further.

Helpful numbers	Telephone number
My maternity hospital is	
My midwife is	
My obstetrician is	
My pharmacist is	
My health visitor is	
My drug/alcohol worker is	
My social worker is	
Other workers involved in my care	

Appendix 5

To access this leaflet as a printable document, please go to www.drugscope.org.uk/pregnancyguide

T-ACE Alcohol screening questionnaire

T-ACE	QUESTIONS	SCORE
Tolerance	How many drinks did it take to make you feel high (to feel the effects of alcohol) before pregnancy? 3 or more = 2 points	
Annoyed	Have people ever annoyed you by criticising your drinking? yes = 1 point	
Cut down	Do you sometimes feel the need to cut down on your drinking? yes = 1 point	
Eye-opener	Do you sometimes take a drink in the morning when you first get up? yes = 1 point	
	Total score	

Scoring

The minimum score is '0' and the maximum score is '5'. A total score of 2 points or more will correctly identify most pregnant women whose drinking is hazardous, harmful or dependent. Further assessment of alcohol use and alcohol related problems would be required.

Source: Sokol RJ, Martier SS, Ager JW. (1989) The T-ACE questions: Practical prenatal detection of risk drinking. *American Journal of Obstetrics and Gynecology*,160, 4, 863-870.

Name of pregnant woman:

Date of birth:

Test completed by: Date of test:

To access this leaflet as a printable document, please go to www.drugscope.org.uk/pregnancyguide

TWEAK Alcohol screening questionnaire

TWEAK	QUESTIONS	SCORE
Tolerance	How many drinks did it take to make you feel high (to feel the effects of alcohol) before pregnancy? 3 or more = 2 points	
Worry	Have close relatives or friends worried or complained about your drinking in the past year? yes = 2 points	
Eye-opener	Do you sometimes have a drink in the morning when you first get up? yes = 1 point	
Amnesia	Has a friend or family member ever told you about things you said or did while you were drinking that you could not remember? yes = 1 point	
K (Cut Down)	Do you sometimes feel the need to cut down on your drinking? yes = 1 point	
	Total score	

Scoring

The minimum score is '0' and the maximum score is '7'. A total score of 2 points or more will correctly identify most women whose drinking is hazardous, harmful or dependent. Further assessment of alcohol use and alcohol related problems would be required.

Source: Russell M. (1994) New assessment tools for risk drinking during pregnancy: T-ACE, TWEAK and others, *Alcohol Health and Research World*, 18, 1, 55-61.

Name of pregnant woman:

Date of birth:

Test completed by: Date of test:

To access this leaflet as a printable document, please go to www.drugscope.org.uk/pregnancyguide

AUDIT Alcohol screening questionnaire

QUESTION	ANSWER	SCORE
1. How often do you have a drink containing alcohol?	Never (0) Monthly or less (1) Two to four times a month (2) Two to three times a week (3) Four or more times a week (4)	
2. How many drinks containing alcohol do you have on a typical day when you are drinking?	1 or 2 (0) 3 or 4 (1) 5 or 6 (2) 7 to 9 (3) 10 or more (4)	
3. How often do you have six or more drinks on one occasion?	Never (0) Less than monthly (1) Monthly (2) Weekly (3) Daily or almost daily (4)	
4. How often during the last year have you found that you were not able to stop drinking once you had started?	Never (0) Less than monthly (1) Monthly (2) Weekly (3) Daily or almost daily (4)	
5. How often during the last year have you failed to do what was normally expected from you because of drinking?	Never (0) Less than monthly (1) Monthly (2) Weekly (3) Daily or almost daily (4)	
6. How often during the last year have you needed a first drink in the morning to get yourself going after a heavy drinking session?	Never (0) Less than monthly (1) Monthly (2) Weekly (3) Daily or almost daily (4)	
7. How often during the last year have you had a feeling of guilt or remorse after drinking?	Never (0) Less than monthly (1) Monthly (2) Weekly (3) Daily or almost daily (4)	

To access this leaflet as a printable document, please go to www.drugscope.org.uk/pregnancyguide

8. How often during the last year have you been unable to remember what happened the night before because you had been drinking?	Never (0) Less than monthly (1) Monthly (2) Weekly (3) Daily or almost daily (4)	
9. Have you or someone else been injured as a result of your drinking?	No (0) Yes, but not in the last year (2) Yes, during the last year (4)	
10. Has a relative or friend, or a doctor or other health worker been concerned about your drinking, or suggested you cut down?	No (0) Yes, but not in the last year (2) Yes, during the last year (4)	
	Total score	

Scoring

Total scores of 8 or more are indicators of hazardous and harmful alcohol use, as well as possible alcohol dependence.

A score of 1 or more on Question 2 or Question 3 indicates consumption at a hazardous or harmful level, and is above recommended level of alcohol consumption for pregnant women.

Points scored above '0' on Questions 4-6 (especially weekly or daily symptoms) indicate signs of alcohol dependence.

Points scored on Questions 7-10 indicate that alcohol-related harm is already being experienced.

Name of pregnant woman:

Date of birth:

Test completed by: Date of test:

Source: Babor TF., Higgins-Biddle JC., Saunders JB., & Monteiro MG.(2001) *AUDIT the alcohol use disorders identification test: guidelines for use in primary care,* 2nd Edition, Geneva, Department of Mental Health and Substance Dependence, World Health Organisation.

Appendix 6

To access this leaflet as a printable document, please go to www.drugscope.org.uk/pregnancyguide

Diary Alcohol and drug use

Day	Times	Type of drug/ drink taken	Amount taken	Where? Why? Effects?

Name: Date:

Appendix 7

To access this leaflet as a printable document, please go to www.drugscope.org.uk/pregnancyguide

Guidance on the use of drug testing (toxicology screening) within the context of child protection practice
Information for health and social care professionals

Introduction

Healthcare services are frequently asked by partner agencies to provide toxicology screening and reports regarding mothers and fathers (including prospective parents) about whom there are concerns related to parenting capacity and child welfare. There is concern about the inappropriate use, inaccurate interpretation, and inadequate reporting and management of such tests.

This guidance aims to provide useful information and advice for health and social care practitioners involved with substance-using parents, regarding the following:
- the clinical use of drug testing for the purposes of drug treatment
- what drug test results indicate and how they should be interpreted
- what drug test results DO NOT indicate
- the limitations of drug testing
- the reporting and management of drug test results by professionals
- the potential role of drug testing, if any, within the context of child care and child protection practice.

Please note: This guidance does not refer to the drug testing of infants and children for forensic and/or diagnostic purposes.

The clinical use of drug testing for the purposes of drug treatment

Illicit, prescribed and over-the-counter drugs and medications can be detected in certain biological samples (e.g. urine, oral fluid, blood and hair) using different testing methods. Many licit and illicit drugs can be inappropriately used, but not all can be identified by routine screening. Drug tests generally target commonly used drugs or drug groups. Procedures for drug testing depend on local drug service requirements and available resources.

Toxicology screening is normally carried out using either urine or oral swabs. Blood and hair testing are not usually carried out by NHS drug services, although they are sometimes used for forensic purposes.

To access this leaflet as a printable document, please go to www.drugscope.org.uk/pregnancyguide

The Department of Health (2007) provides clinical guidelines on the use of drug testing (toxicology screening) for the purposes of drug treatment.

Drug testing is a clinical tool which can assist decision-making regarding drug treatment. For example:

- As part of the assessment process, to confirm the patient is taking drugs
- To inform decisions regarding drug treatment, such as substitute prescribing
- To help establish the efficacy of, and compliance with, drug treatment over a period of time
- As part of the review process, to help confirm that the patient is taking their prescribed medication
- To help monitor illicit drug use, including as a drug-specific treatment goal (for example, as part of a psychosocial intervention or detoxification programme)
- To support honest dialogue between clinician and patient regarding progress on treatment.

Drug tests can also be used for quality assurance purposes and requirements.

Decisions about drug treatment are never made solely on the basis of a drug test. Drug screen results are used as a clinical guide and treatment measure and are not intended to be used punitively. Coercive measures to obtain drug tests and punitive responses to positive drug test results may deter patients from attending health and social care appointments, resulting in poorer outcomes. Equally, it is important to ensure that the needs of patients, whose test results show no apparent problems, are not overlooked.

Drug testing is always performed with the patient's knowledge and informed consent. Department of Health (2007) guidelines state that random and intermittent drug screening 'is probably the most practical and cost-effective option for providing reliable information about an individual's recent drug use'. Drug testing to confirm illicit drug use when a patient has admitted to it, and is already in treatment, is generally NOT cost-effective.

Please note: The rationale for testing and the use made of test results is important and must be understood by those responsible for patient care in order to be effective.

To access this leaflet as a printable document, please go to www.drugscope.org.uk/pregnancyguide

---

What drug test results indicate and how they should be interpreted

Toxicology screening can detect the presence or absence of certain types of drugs and their metabolites. Oral swab and urine drug screen results simply indicate 'positive' or 'negative' for each drug type, or 'undetermined' for a specific reason.

The following drugs and drug groups are normally included in toxicology screens:
- methadone
- other opiates
- cocaine
- amphetamines
- benzodiazepines.

Cannabis is *not* usually included and toxicology screening does *not* detect alcohol.

Please note: Department of Health (2007) guidelines emphasise that drug test results should always be interpreted within the context in which they were taken and in the light of other clinical information. This might include current prescribing (if any), information given by the patient regarding non-prescribed drug use, stage of drug treatment, and the patient's personal and social circumstances.

What drug test results DO NOT indicate*
- Drug tests do not measure the quantities of drug taken
- Drug tests do not measure frequency of use (e.g. sporadic or continuous)
- Drug tests do not measure drug tolerance levels
- Drug tests do not confirm or measure drug dependence or drug dependence severity
- Drug tests do not pinpoint the precise time drugs are taken (only a "window period" – which varies depending on the drug type, dose, pattern of consumption, route of administration, and test sample)
- More importantly, drug tests do not indicate whether the drugs taken had any significant effect on the person's mental state or behaviour.

Drug tests do not distinguish between drug use and problem drug use**. Positive drug test results for illicit drugs do not establish that the use of the drug/s resulted

---

* Relates to oral swab and urine toxicology screening.
** Problem drug use means drug use with serious negative consequences of a physical, psychological, social and interpersonal, financial or legal nature for users and those around them. Such drug use is usually heavy, with features of dependence, and typically involves use of one or more of the following: heroin, other opiates, benzodiazepines, cocaine, amphetamines (ACMD 2003).

To access this leaflet as a printable document, please go to www.drugscope.org.uk/pregnancyguide

in adverse consequences for the individual or those around them. A positive result does not necessarily indicate that treatment is needed, or required.

Equally, *negative* test results for illicit drugs do not necessarily indicate that an individual:
- is using their prescribed drugs as directed,
- is not adversely affected by their drug-taking behaviour, and
- is not using illicit drugs or alcohol intermittently or perhaps regularly.

The limitations of drug testing

There are a number of limitations to drug testing procedures and analysis which need to be taken into account.

Detection windows and the sensitivity of different drug tests can result in false positive and false negative results.

Some over-the-counter medications can result in positive screens. For example, over-the-counter drugs which contain codeine or dihydrocodeine preparations can result in positive opiate results. Tests to differentiate which opiate has been taken are sometimes required.

Samples can be prone to problems of adulteration, substitution, non-compliance and pre-collection abstinence, producing misleading results (Department of Health 2007). For example, ingestion of certain drugs obtained licitly (e.g. prescribed methadone, dihydrocodeine and diazepam) may mask those taken illicitly.

It is advised that confirmatory testing is requested if the result is unexpected or contested, or if substantial weight is to be placed on the result. Confirmatory testing is essential for forensic purposes such as testing in relation to court orders or sentences, and when test results may have serious consequences for patients or their families – for example, in relation to drug management or child protection (Department of Health 2007).

The reporting and management of drug test results by professionals

Department of Health (2007) guidelines state that it should be normal practice to have written procedures for drug testing, including the discussion and management of reported results.

To access this leaflet as a printable document, please go to www.drugscope.org.uk/pregnancyguide

Drug testing should be conducted *when clinically indicated* and when deemed appropriate by the *clinician responsible for the patient's clinical drug management plan*, in accordance with service requirements and standards of care.

Discussion of drug test results and responses to positive and negative test results need to be individually tailored, and consistent with the clinical drug management plan. Practitioners responsible for patient care are advised to ensure that drug test results are *only* provided to non-clinical services as part of a comprehensive account of the patient's drug-taking history, reported drug-taking behaviour, drug treatment progress and drug treatment plan.

The *rationale for testing* and the *use made of drug test results* must be clearly explained. Professionals involved in the care of a family should ensure that this information is documented.

The potential role of drug testing, if any, within the context of child care and child protection practice

Drug test results *on their own*, do not provide 'evidence' of adequate or inadequate parenting capacity or child care. The value of drug testing in determining the effects of parental drug use on parenting capacity is therefore limited, especially in the absence of more robust forms of parenting capacity and child welfare assessment procedures and processes. Taken out of context, toxicology results provide a relatively crude and potentially misleading indicator of progress and should not, *on their own*, be used to 'substantiate' parenting capacity or child welfare assessments or decision-making regarding the safeguarding and protection of children. Instead, practitioners are advised to refer to agreed child protection procedures and good practice guidelines.

Whilst Department of Health (2007:16) guidelines refer to the possibility of drug test results being used within the context of child protection practice, there are currently no agreed policies or protocols, standards or competency frameworks to guide such practice. This presents a challenge in terms of governance, as well as organisational and professional responsibility and accountability. Within this context, individual practitioners must be satisfied that they are able to explain, demonstrate and defend their practice where necessary.

Please note: Department of Health (2007) guidelines advise that all staff who perform, interpret, and manage drug tests should be sufficiently trained and competent to do so.

THE ESSENTIAL **Guide to Problem Substance Use During Pregnancy**

Appendix 8

To access this leaflet as a printable document, please go to www.drugscope.org.uk/pregnancyguide

Neonatal Abstinence Syndrome assessment score chart

Unit no:

Name:

Date of birth:

Birth weight:

Gestational age:

Please fill in score for each 4 hour period.

Write score for each symptom and add together for total score.

If no symptoms enter score = 0

Insert date at beginning of each day and enter [23/06] [2 pm]
time at the beginning of each 4 hour period e.g.

Scoring Mild symptoms = 0-5 Moderate symptoms = 6-13 Severe symptoms = 14-21

Information for parents If baby has a seizure (fit), dial 999 for an ambulance. If baby has moderate to severe symptoms, seek advice and help from your midwife, GP or hospital.

Symptom:	Score:	Date											
		Time											
Feeding	Not able to feed at all	4											
	Demands hourly feeds	2											
	Feeds very slowly (takes more than 30 minutes)	2											
Weight from Day 7 onwards	Loss	4											
	Same	2											
	Gain	0											
	Under 7 days old	0											
Condition of bottom	Raw/broken skin	3											
	Very red	2											
	Mild red	1											
Resting/ sleeping after feeds	Less than 1 hour	5											
	1-2 hours	3											
	2-3 hours	1											
Crying/ irritability	All the time	5											
	Most of the time	4											
	Only some of the time	1											
	Total score													
Drug treatment													
Start time or change dose													

Comments

Appendix 9

To access this leaflet as a printable document, please go to www.drugscope.org.uk/pregnancyguide

Caring for a baby with drug withdrawal symptoms

Information for Parents

This leaflet provides you with information and advice that will help you prepare for the arrival of your baby. Hopefully after reading this you will:
- feel well-informed about baby withdrawals
- understand what your baby might need
- feel confident about how to take care of your baby.

Drugs and the newborn baby

Most drugs (including tobacco and alcohol) that you take when you are pregnant pass through the placenta and are absorbed by your baby.

If a mother is *dependent* or 'addicted' to certain drugs, the baby will have been exposed to these drugs during pregnancy and may develop *withdrawal symptoms* after birth. The medical name for baby withdrawal symptoms is **'Neonatal Abstinence Syndrome'**.

Unfortunately, there is no way of telling exactly how a baby will react as there are many different factors that affect withdrawal symptoms in babies. This is why we like to prepare all parents just in case. What we can say is that drug withdrawal in babies is now fairly common, so you are not alone.

Baby withdrawal symptoms occur quite often with:
- opiate drugs (e.g. methadone, heroin, dihydrocodeine, buprenorphine)
- benzodiazepine drugs (e.g. diazepam and temazepam), and
- heavy alcohol use.

If your baby does develop withdrawal symptoms, these are usually easily managed and the baby will recover in time. Most infants affected by withdrawal symptoms achieve normal growth and development by around 6 months of age and suffer no long term harm, if they are cared for properly.

To access this leaflet as a printable document, please go to www.drugscope.org.uk/pregnancyguide

Midwives and other maternity staff as well as health visitors and GPs have experience in looking after babies and can offer good advice and help to parents.

How babies are affected

Baby withdrawal symptoms are similar to how adults feel when they suddenly stop drinking or stop taking drugs (go 'cold turkey'). However, there are important differences between the way adults are affected and the way babies are affected.

Withdrawal symptoms in babies vary a lot. You might expect to see some or all of the following symptoms:

- high-pitched crying
- excessive (long-lasting) crying
- irritability (easily disturbed or upset)
- sleeping difficulties (the baby cannot settle or sleep after a feed)
- feeding difficulties (the baby is often keen to feed but cannot suck or swallow properly)
- vomiting (unable to keep milk down)
- diarrhoea (frequent loose stools or runny poos)
- a sore red bottom (due to frequent dirty nappies)
- poor weight gain or weight loss
- restlessness (unable to lie still for any length of time)
- tremor (shakiness) and jitteriness
- skin abrasions (sores from moving around a lot)
- stuffy nose and sneezing
- rapid breathing
- fever (a high temperature).

Occasionally, babies have convulsions (fits) but this is very rare.

Most babies who have been exposed to drugs before birth will have some symptoms after birth. Some babies have only *mild* withdrawal symptoms and require no more than the usual care that all babies need. Other babies have more *severe* symptoms where they might not be able to feed or sleep properly and they lose weight rather than gain weight. These babies usually need special care at home or in hospital (the 'neonatal unit' or 'special care baby unit') and may need calming drugs to help them recover. Some babies can be irritable for weeks or months, but symptoms gradually improve with time.

To access this leaflet as a printable document, please go to www.drugscope.org.uk/pregnancyguide

It is important to remember that babies with withdrawal symptoms can have difficulty responding in the normal way to their carers. This is because of the way the withdrawal symptoms affect the baby's functioning. Certain forms of parent-infant contact and supportive comfort measures have been shown to help babies who have withdrawal symptoms (see pages 4-5). If your baby develops withdrawal symptoms, you will be given more advice on these. We suggest that you follow this advice so you can care for your baby confidently.

Assessing babies to see if they have withdrawals

Withdrawal symptoms in babies can begin within a few hours of birth, or as late as 10 days after, but most babies who develop withdrawals show signs within 24-72 hours after birth. Mothers who are dependent on drugs and/or alcohol are therefore asked to stay in hospital (in the postnatal ward) with their baby for at least 3 days (72 hours).

In the postnatal ward mothers are expected to care for their baby at all times and are encouraged to bond with their baby and breastfeed. Mothers and babies are not separated unless this is absolutely necessary – for example, if the baby is really unwell. Normally, a score chart is used to assess the condition of the baby and parents are shown how to use it. Withdrawal symptoms in babies can be similar to other conditions and medical problems so it is important to make a proper assessment. The assessment involves keeping a close eye on the baby, scoring certain signs and symptoms and writing down how severe each symptom is over a period of time.

Most babies can go home after 3 days (even if they develop symptoms), where they can be cared for by their parents, with the help and support of the midwife, health visitor and GP. Most babies need some special care and attention for a while afterwards, and the midwife, health visitor and GP will want to check on how well the baby is feeding, sleeping, putting on weight and responding to you and its environment.

Some babies can become unwell *after* they are discharged home. This is because some drugs (like benzodiazepines such as 'valium') can take longer to leave the baby's system. Parents are encouraged to keep a close eye on their baby and to continue using the score chart for at least a week after leaving hospital.

Babies admitted to the neonatal unit

If a baby develops *severe* withdrawal symptoms they might be admitted to the 'neonatal unit' or 'special care baby unit'. Here they can get 'tube' feeds and calming medicine if necessary. Treatment and care aims to reduce the baby's distress and discomfort and to get the baby feeding and sleeping as normally as possible. Babies usually stay in the neonatal unit for about 10 days, but occasionally for longer. Most admissions to the neonatal unit happen when the baby is still in hospital after birth, but babies are also admitted from home. If the baby's problems get worse at home then it is better to admit the baby earlier rather than later. This is why we are keen to offer parents extra help at home and to see how the baby is doing.

Tips on caring for your baby

If your baby does develop withdrawal symptoms, we know from experience, and through research, that there are certain things that tend to help the baby recover.

Here are some suggestions:

Crying and irritability
- Make sure your baby is kept in a quiet room and has calm surroundings - no bright lights or loud sounds that might upset your baby and make them more irritable.
- Handle your baby gently and as little as possible - this will reduce the level of stimulation and will keep your baby calmer.
- Use a dummy or pacifier ('soothers')... unless you are breastfeeding.
- If your baby has a lot of 'skin-to-skin' contact, they will cry less.
- Try giving your baby a very gentle massage.
- Humming, singing softly or gently rocking your baby may help.

Feeding problems
- Feed your baby in a quiet place with minimal disruption.
- Feed your baby on demand - frequent small feeds are normally better.
- Allow time for resting in between sucking.
- Burp your baby very gently when they stop sucking and after the feed.
- Gently support your baby's cheeks and lower jaw to help improve their efforts to suck and swallow.

To access this leaflet as a printable document, please go to www.drugscope.org.uk/pregnancyguide

- If your baby has a lot of 'skin-to-skin' contact, the baby will feed better.
- Try giving your baby a very gentle tummy massage.
- Keep a record of all the feeds your baby takes so that the midwife or health visitor can check whether your baby is feeding well enough, getting enough calories, and putting on enough weight.

Sleeping problems

- Let your baby sleep in a quiet room, with minimal disturbance. Keep the room dim (no bright lights) and try not to pat or touch your baby too much.
- Make sure your baby has a clean dry nappy – check for nappy rash and apply hospital formula nappy rash cream or zinc cream if needed.
- Make sure your baby has clean bedding and clothes which are free from vomit. The smell of vomit may make your baby sick again and vomit may irritate their delicate skin.
- Soft, gentle music, humming or gently rocking your baby may help.
- Avoid getting your baby too hot.
- Never smoke in the same room (or house) as your baby.

Movement problems

- Swaddle your baby (by snugly wrapping the baby up in a soft blanket) – this may help to comfort your baby and to stop too much movement.
- Keep your baby in a warm quiet room.
- Use soft flannel blankets or a short-haired sheep skin covered by a cotton sheet for the baby's comfort.
- Avoid handling your baby too much if it is very restless, jittery or trembling – keep any stimulation down to a minimum to help calm the baby.

Skin problems

- Regularly check and change your baby's nappy.
- Change your baby's clothes frequently, especially if they sweat a lot.
- Cover your baby's hands with gloves or mittens if skin becomes damaged from too much fist sucking.
- Keep any areas of damaged skin clean – avoid baby lotions as your baby may suck them.
- To help prevent nappy rash and sores apply hospital formula nappy rash cream or zinc cream around the baby's bottom area.

Breathing problems

- Make sure no one smokes near your baby, ensure there is clean air and the room is warm.
- Keep your baby's nose and mouth clean.
- Feed your baby slowly, allowing rest periods in-between sucking.
- Avoid overdressing or wrapping your baby too tightly.
- Keep your baby in a well supported semi-sitting position, avoid putting the baby on its tummy to sleep.
- Keep a close eye on your baby. If breathing difficulties continue or worsen, contact your GP, midwife or health visitor, or call 999.

Temperature problems

- Keep clothing to a minimum and avoid a lot of bedclothes – avoid getting your baby too hot.
- If your baby has a lot of 'skin-to-skin' contact, this will help to control your baby's body temperature.
- Seek medical help if your baby has a high temperature for more than 4 hours. Call the midwife, health visitor or GP.

Other problems

- If your baby has severe vomiting or diarrhoea and becomes dehydrated, contact your midwife, health visitor, GP or hospital for advice immediately.
- If your baby has a convulsion (fit), dial 999 and ask for an ambulance to take your baby to hospital.

Getting support

It is very important that you get all the help and support you need. Show this leaflet to your partner and any other person (family or friends) who will be supporting you to look after your baby. There are a lot of myths about baby withdrawal symptoms and a lot of bad feelings towards mothers who use alcohol or drugs. Many parents say that they feel guilty and 'to blame' for their baby's condition and find baby withdrawal symptoms a difficult subject to talk about. This is why we like to mention it early on in the pregnancy. This way you can get some reliable information and not feel anxious about your baby.

To access this leaflet as a printable document, please go to www.drugscope.org.uk/pregnancyguide

We know that babies with withdrawal symptoms can be very difficult to look after and they can require a lot of patience and time. Experience has shown us that there are many things that you can do to calm and comfort your baby and to help improve their condition. Even so, if you find that caring for your baby is too stressful, don't be afraid to ask for help from NHS professionals and services. Remember that we are always here to provide you with support and to talk to you about any worries or questions that you may have.

Please feel free to speak with your midwife or other health care professional about the information in this leaflet, especially if there is anything that you don't understand or would like to talk about further. We hope that this leaflet has given you enough information to help you prepare for the arrival of your baby.

Helpful numbers   Telephone number

My maternity hospital is
_____

My midwife is
_____

My obstetrician is
_____

My pharmacist is
_____

My health visitor is
_____

My drug/alcohol worker is
_____

My social worker is
_____

Other workers involved in my care
_____

Appendix 10

To access this leaflet as a printable document, please go to www.drugscope.org.uk/pregnancyguide

ALF1 ## Antenatal Liaison Form (problem substance use)

Mother's name: _____

Date of birth: _____

Address: _____

Postcode: _____

Telephone: _____

Mother's CHI/NHS No: _____

E.D.D: _____

Date attended booking: _____

Parity: _____

Consultant obstetrician: _____ Tel: _____

Midwife: _____ Tel: _____

GP: _____ Tel: _____

Health visitor: _____ Tel: _____

Drug/alcohol worker: _____ Tel: _____

Social worker: _____ Tel: _____

Other support worker: _____ Tel: _____

Details of substance use

Tobacco use? Yes ☐ No ☐ If yes, number per day? _____

Alcohol use? (average weekly consumption 1st trimester)

0 units ☐   1-7 units ☐   8-21 units ☐   22-42 units ☐   > 42 units ☐

To access this leaflet as a printable document, please go to www.drugscope.org.uk/pregnancyguide

Pattern of alcohol use? e.g. drinking >3 units every day, binge drinking (>5 units in one occasion)

Evidence of alcohol dependence? e.g. withdrawal symptoms, tolerance, daily intoxication etc

Attending Specialist Alcohol Treatment Service? Yes ☐ No ☐

Name of specialist service:

Tel:

Prescribed substitute medication for drug dependence at booking
(enter drugs & daily dosage)

Name of prescriber: Tel:

Pharmacy: Tel:

Dispensing arrangements (e.g. daily pick up/twice weekly/3 x weekly/supervised consumption)

Previous pregnancy affected by **maternal** problem drug/alcohol use?
Yes ☐ No ☐

Previous baby affected by Neonatal Abstinence Syndrome/Fetal Alcohol Syndrome?
Yes ☐ No ☐

Referred to specialist midwife/pregnancy service?
Yes ☐ No ☐

Illicit (street) drug use since conception?

(Enter all drugs used during pregnancy, *excluding those prescribed*)
Answer YES or NO

YES/NO		Drug used
☐	☐	Heroin
☐	☐	Cannabis
☐	☐	Methadone (street supply)
☐	☐	Cocaine / Crack
☐	☐	Dihydrocodeine (street supply)
☐	☐	Amphetamine ('speed')
☐	☐	Buprenorphine e.g. Subutex or Suboxone (street supply)
☐	☐	Ecstasy
☐	☐	Diazepam (street supply)
☐	☐	Volatile substances e.g. gas/glue

Other opiates – please state _____

Other stimulants – please state _____

Other tranquillizer – please state _____

Over the counter drugs – please state _____

Other drug use – please state _____

Injecting drug use?

Ever injected drugs? Yes ☐ No ☐

Ever injected drugs during pregnancy? Yes ☐ No ☐

If yes, date of last injection? _____

If yes, frequency of injecting? e.g. every day/once weekly etc) _____

List drugs injected during pregnancy e.g. heroin, cocaine

_____

_____

To access this leaflet as a printable document, please go to www.drugscope.org.uk/pregnancyguide

Attending Specialist Drug Treatment Service?   Yes ☐ No ☐

Name of service: Tel:

Blood Borne Viruses – Antenatal testing for:

HIV   test accepted ☐ declined ☐ result_____

Hepatitis B   test accepted ☐ declined ☐ result_____

HBV immunised?   Yes ☐ No ☐

Hepatitis C   test offered? Yes ☐ No ☐

If yes,   accepted ☐ declined ☐ result_____

Father's/ partner's name:

Address:

Date of Birth: Tel:

GP: Tel:

Tobacco / alcohol / drug use of partner? – please detail consumption

Prescribed substitute medication?

Partner's HIV / hepatitis B / hepatitis C status? (if known)

Form completed by:

Date form completed:

To access this leaflet as a printable document, please go to www.drugscope.org.uk/pregnancyguide

ALF1

Complete at 32 week appointment

Update
Antenatal Liaison Form (problem substance use)

Mother's name: _____ Date of birth: _____

Address: _____

Postcode: _____ Tel: _____

Hospital unit number _____ Mother's CHI/NHS No: _____

E.D.D: _____

Changes to named professionals?

Consultant obstetrician: _____ Tel: _____

Midwife: _____ Tel: _____

GP: _____ Tel: _____

Health visitor: _____ Tel: _____

Drug/alcohol worker: _____ Tel: _____

Social worker: _____ Tel: _____

Other support worker: _____ Tel: _____

Changes to *prescribed* drugs during pregnancy? (record any medication/dose changes and date of change)

_____

_____

_____

Change of pharmacy? add new details (address and telephone number) and date of change

_____

_____

To access this leaflet as a printable document, please go to www.drugscope.org.uk/pregnancyguide

Change in illicit (street) drug use? Please detail

Change in alcohol consumption? Please detail

Change in tobacco consumption? Please detail

Additional information regarding father? Please detail

PLF1

Complete on
May 10. Send
copy to GP
and health
visitor

Postnatal Liaison Form (problem substance use)

Mother's name: _____   Date of birth: _____

Address: _____

_____

Father's name: _____   Father's d.o.b: _____

Address: _____

Baby's name: _____

Address: _____

Mother's Unit No: _____   Mother's CHI/NHS No.: _____

Baby's SM number: _____   Baby's CHI/NHS No.: _____

Pregnancy outcome details:

Delivery date: _____

Gestation: _____   APGARs: _____

Birth weight: _____   Cord pH: _____

Birth length: _____   Head Circumference: _____

Labour ward (please provide details... if none state 'none')

Mode of delivery? _____

Complications in labour? _____

Pain relief during labour? _____

Complications of delivery? _____

Problems at birth? _____

To access this leaflet as a printable document, please go to www.drugscope.org.uk/pregnancyguide

Postnatal ward

Baby stayed for 72 hours observation?   Yes ☐ No ☐

Neonatal withdrawal symptoms developed within 72 hours?   Yes ☐ No ☐

If yes, severity?   mild ☐ moderate ☐ severe ☐

Drug treatment administered?

Medication on discharge?

Breast or bottle feeding on discharge?

Other comments?

Postnatal discharge date:

Neonatal Unit

Admission date:

Reason for admission:

Neonatal withdrawal symptoms?   None ☐ Mild ☐ Moderate ☐ Severe ☐

Drug treatment administered for NAS?

Medication on discharge?

Breast or bottle feeding on discharge?

Other comments?

Neonatal Unit discharge date:

Community

Baby developed NAS symptoms *after* discharge from hospital?   Yes ☐ No ☐

If yes, symptoms   Mild ☐ Moderate ☐ Severe ☐

Baby readmitted?   Neonatal Unit ☐   Children's Ward ☐

Date of admission:

Date of discharge:

To access this leaflet as a printable document, please go to www.drugscope.org.uk/pregnancyguide

---

Infant feeding at day 10?   Breast fed ☐   Bottle fed ☐

Continued drug/alcohol use whilst breastfeeding? (please list all drugs taken and amounts)

_____

_____

_____

Paediatric follow-up of baby required?   Yes ☐   No ☐

If yes, state reason: _____

_____

Form completed by: _____

Date form completed: _____

Named community midwife: _____

Team: _____   Tel: _____

Name of health visitor: _____   Tel: _____

Address: _____

_____

Name of GP: _____   Tel: _____

Address: _____

_____

Appendix 11

To access this leaflet as a printable document, please go to www.drugscope.org.uk/pregnancyguide

Assignment for allocation of GP

FAO: Primary Care Services

Address:

Date:

Please allocate me a new general practitioner. My details are below.

Surname:

First name:

Previous surname:

Date of Birth: Gender: Male ☐   Female ☐

CHI/NHS Number (if known):

Present address (include postcode):

Previous address (include postcode):

Name, address and telephone number of previous GP (if none, state reason why):

Names of GP practices that have refused to accept me as a patient:

Other family members who require to be assigned (list their full name, date of birth, and gender). Use a separate sheet of paper if required.

I declare that the information I have given on this letter is correct and complete. I understand that I am only entitled to be registered with one GP practice at any given time in order to receive general medical services.

Signature:

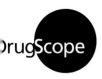

What is DrugScope ?

DrugScope is the UK's leading independent centre of expertise on drugs and the national membership organisation for the drug field. Our aim is to inform policy development, reduce drug-related harms to individuals, families and communities – and promote health, well-being, recovery, inclusion and integration. We provide quality drug information, promote effective responses to drug taking, undertake research, advise on policy-making, encourage informed debate – particularly in the media – and speak for our member organisations working on the ground.

What does DrugScope do?

DrugScope's objectives are:

   to provide a national voice for the drug sector
   to inform policy development drawing on the experience and expertise of our members
   to work with others to develop 'joined up' responses to drug and alcohol problems
   to support drug services and promote good practice
   to improve public understanding of drugs and drug policy.

DrugScope represents the views and concerns of our members to Ministers, officials, MPs and Peers, the media and others. We create opportunities for informed debate through regional and national forums, conferences and seminars. For more about our work, please visit www.drugscope.org.uk

Who are our members?

Drug and alcohol problems impact on the work of practitioners and organisations across health, social care, criminal justice, housing and related areas. DrugScope has around 600 members – individuals and organisations – working in adult and young people's treatment, service managers and commissioners, children and young people's services, drug education and related sectors including healthcare, social work, housing and criminal justice.

Our members receive 6 issues of *Druglink* magazine and 12 issues of *Members' briefing* each year, as well as invitations to regional and national member consultation events and fora, discounts on DrugScope publications and conferences and free copies of DrugScope reports and briefings. Membership starts from as little as £60 per year. To find out more about membership, please visit our website at: www.drugscope.org.uk/membership

Druglink magazine

DrugScope publishes *Druglink*, a bi-monthly magazine for all those UK professionals interested in drugs and drug-related issues – whether it's treatment, public health, education and prevention, criminal justice or international. *Druglink* includes the latest news, feature articles, interviews, factsheets, reviews and listings. To find out more, please visit our website at: http://www.drugscope.org.uk/publications/druglink

DrugScope publications

The Essential Series is DrugScope's range of resource books for professionals who work with drug users. The publications catalogue can be viewed at www.drugscope.org.uk/publications/catalogue

The Essential Guide to Drugs and Alcohol (2010)

With half a million copies sold since its launch in 1982 and now in its 14th edition, The Essential Guide to Drugs and Alcohol is indispensable to everyone with a professional interest in the field. With an A-Z of illicit substances including new sections on BZP, mephedrone and naphyrone, a jargon buster of key sector terms and accessible tables on seizure stats and prevalence, the guide pulls together complex information in an easily digestible way. The book is available to order from HIT for £14.95 (0844 412 0972 / www.hit.org.uk)